From the Couch to Katahdin

By DerinDuo
a/k/a
Colleen & Rex Derin

TheDerinDuo@yahoo.com

From the Couch to Katahdin

Homemade in the USA!

Photography by Rex Derin
Graphic Art work by Colleen Derin

CONTENTS

introduction   (i) - (iii)

Special Thanks to: (iv)

Chapter 1.   page   1

Chapter 2.   page   4

Chapter 3.   page 30

Chapter 4.   page 37

Chapter 5.   page 55

Chapter 6.   page 60

Chapter 7.   page 63

Chapter 8.   page 74

Chapter 9.   page 88

Chapter 10.   page 93

and finally,   page 103

INTRODUCTION

Before we get started,
this section contains:
history, terms used, and a giggle.

What is the Appalachian Trail?

It is the world's longest continuous mountain trail. It measures approximately 2183 miles extending from Mt Katahdin in Maine to Springer Mountain in Georgia.

The trail is marked by using white blazes (stripes) which are roughly 6 inches long and 2 inches wide.

The trail goes thru 14 states: Maine, New Hampshire, Vermont, Massachusetts, Connecticut, New Jersey, New York, Pennsylvania, Maryland, Virginia, West Virginia, North Carolina, Tennessee, and Georgia.

The history of the Appalachian Trail in 4 sentences:

It was the idea of a forester, Benton Mackeye in 1921 that gave birth to the Appalachian Trail. The first section of the trail, from Bear Mountain west through Harriman State Park to Arden, New York, was first opened October 7th, 1923. Mackaye then called for a two-day Appalachian Trail conference to be held in March 1925 in Washington, D.C. which in turn gave birth to The Appalachian Trail Conservancy. The trail kept growing and Earl Shaffer of Pennsylvania was the first thru-hiker in 1948.

Eighty percent of those who attempt to complete the trail never do. Three quarters of the A.T. hikers are men. There were 44 couples that completed the trail last year.

There are blue blazes leading off the white blazed trail that lead to lean-tos or shelters or it may be a short cut and less physically demanding trail.

If an A. T. hiker is said to be "blue blazing", it means that he is cheating on the actual A.T. (white blazed) trail.

Slack packing is when a hiker leaves his pack with someone who will give it back to him further down the trail so that the hiker doesn't have to carry it.

A no-bo is a north bound hiker.

A so-bo is a south bound hiker.

A flip flop is a hike that starts from one end or area and then jumps to another end or area to complete the whole trail. Sometimes this is done for weather reasons.

By strict definition a "thru hike" takes 12 months or less.

A section hiker does parts or all of the trail by sections.

"Yogi bearing" is a term used to describe a hiker that tries to get food (mainly) from day hikers or families visiting the trail.

A hostel is where a hiker can spend the night either by paying for it or not. There is generally a food supply of some type at a hostel.

Trail Magic is a kind gesture to a hiker or perhaps an unexpected bonus of some sort.

The hiker may know who has helped him/her in some way but most times he doesn't know. The person performing the Trail Magic is known as a Trail Angel.

Common examples of Trail Magic are:
a ride into town, to buy new boots, or to a Doctor
food or water or beverages that is either left along the trail
or given directly to the hiker
There are many interesting stories about Trail Magic.

for your amusement:

The first hiker is a day hiker and he goes past some spilt M & M candies on the trail and he steps over them.

The second hiker is a section hiker and he goes past some spilt M & M candies on the trail and he admires their pretty colors and considers snatching them up.

The third hiker, a "thru hiker" sees the spilt candies and yells "yippee! Trail Magic!".

Special Thanks to:

God, we couldn't have done it without you.

My husband, for too many reasons to list.

To our families and friends for their moral support.

To Joe and Mina, our kitty nannies, for watching our home, bringing in the mail, taking care of our vehicles, feeding and playing with the kitties, and last but not least; litter scooping.

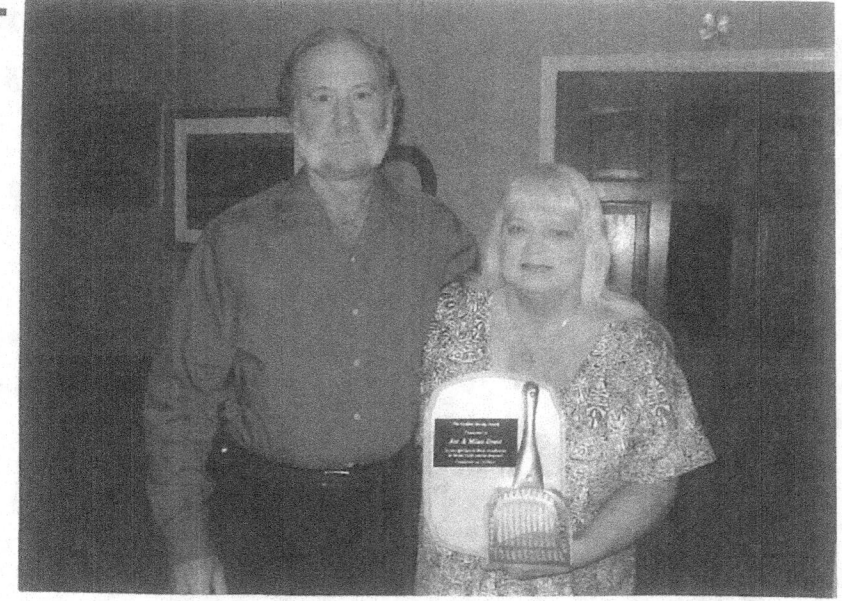

Joe and Mina have been awarded the Golden Scoop Award for "Excellence in Fecal Matter Removal"

Last, but certainly not least. Thank you to the trail maintenance crews and to the ridge runners who act as the "neighborhood watch" and report to the maintenance crews or authorities if needed.

Chapter 1

June 2010 Getting Ready for Trail

Well our adventure begins in one calendar month. Oh boy! We have so much to do and we have been preparing for months. We been researching by meeting up with those who have done hiking. They have passed along some of their knowledge and allowed us to see and handle their gear. We have met up with a man here in Titusville who has written an A.T. guide book. We have purchased numerous books, videos and magazines in order to better prepare ourselves.

We have been breaking in our hiking boots and shoes. We have changed our bank from a local credit union to a much larger bank that has on-line software with which I am familiar using. Now, I am setting up all of our accounts to be paid online. I think that we are prepared.

It has been just barely over one year since I was in the hospital from a heart attack on the night of my divorce. Now, I am happily remarried and my stress level is normal. I haven't had a passing out spell in about a year either. The heart doctor told me that I had "broken heart syndrome" from the stress of my divorce and that the heart catheterization didn't show any blockages large enough to stint. So, we have both had numerous doctor visits. We have had blood tests, x-rays, and I have Epipens, nitroglycerine, antihistamines, antibiotics and Prednisone. I still need a couple of things for our emergency kit.

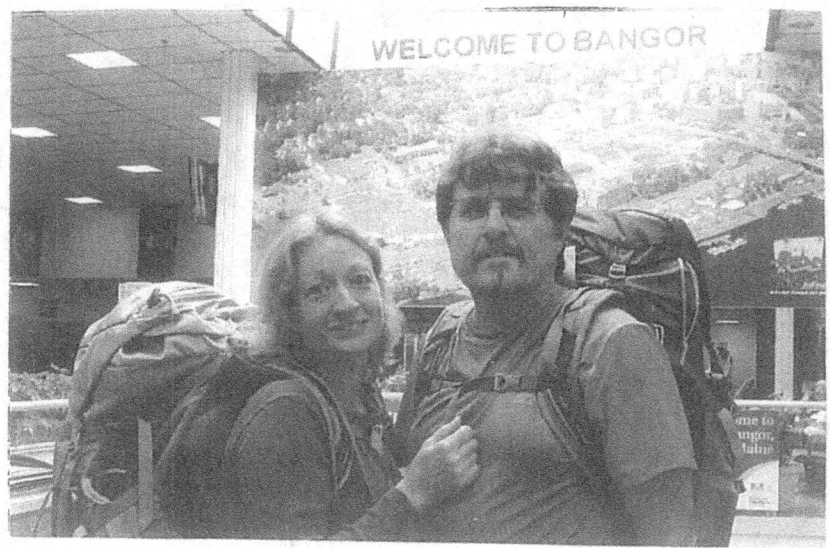

We are ready to go.

Getting the Jitters

O.K. I am in between flipping out and being really excited! So much to remember. So many things to do in preparation.

Many people have had interesting things to tell us; like one couple's daughter who has done the hike and the experiences that she had. More people than I realized have hiked at least a portion of it. Those that have first hand experience always have a certain look on their faces when they tell us about "their Hike". I intend on taking lots of pictures of "our hike". So, with out having to pay for a morning newspaper, computer access and cable TV, no gas expenses for the car, and car insurance on suspension, financially; we should be doing well! Lets pray our health does o.k. and we can tent camp the whole way. As many have told me "this is the chance of a lifetime". I have to agree.

As the daughter of an English teacher I feel badly not going over and over these journal entries and making sure that they are grammatically correct. Perhaps this is the first step of my journey! "Let go" and "Lets go"! Thanks for bearing with me.

POST TRAIL UPDATE:

Nothing that we did to prepare ourselves helped.

The bills still got all screwed up in ways that are unimaginable.

We did save money in the ways that I listed above however the trail cost us *way* more than we ever thought. In the trails defense, we could have spent less but for us the trail is not about who suffers the most.

Hows this work again?

This book contains actual blogs that were written on the trail. I (Colleen) wrote most of the blogs. The ones that Rex wrote and helped co-write are towards the beginning. Typing is not easy for Rex and computers can be extra hard on him.

Sometimes the writing will be out of chronological order or go back and forth in time because as a hiker making live blogs it can be difficult to know what you have already written about with everything running thru your head or there are so many things that you remember later to include.

Getting actual computer time is very challenging also.

So, hold onto your hiking poles....here we go!

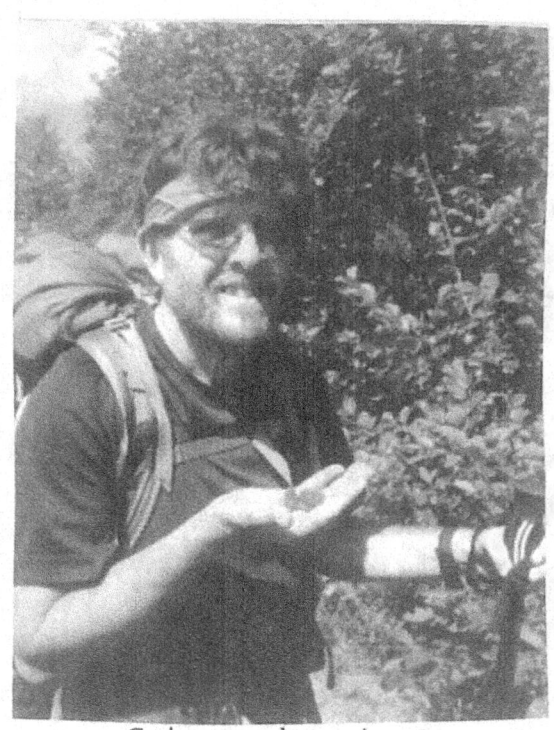

Got raspberries?

CHAPTER 2
AND OFF WE GO.......

We flew up to Bangor Maine with intentions of taking a bus to Millinocket and from there we would find a way to Baxter State Park. We made reservations to spend 3 nights at Baxter. The first night was just to get there and settled in. The second day we'd climb Mt. Katahdin, and I gave us an extra day for anything unforeseen and in case our legs had gotten real sore.

It was just a couple weeks prior to our departure date that we learned that the bus from the airport only goes to Millinocket once a day and the schedule was not going to work for us. So, we called (our first) hostel owners who provided shuttle service. I apologized to the woman on the phone that we had not made arrangements to stay with her. We had read about her place but we were trying to save our nickels. Not a problem, she'd come pick us up and take us to Baxter State Park. She was right at the airport on time when we arrived and picked us up just like family. We climbed into her SUV with our packs and we each had a separate bag for things that wouldn't fit in our packs. As she was driving she gently mentioned that we were carrying a lot of gear.

She said that her husband was especially good at helping people get their pack weights down. We knew that we had "a little" extra weight but once I'd figured out which shoes I'd be wearing I could mail back home the others. She asked how many pairs did I have? I told her that I had a pair of hiking boots, a pair of lower cut hiking shoes, flip flops for around camp, and water shoes for where we had to ford water. She seemed to think that it was a whole lot of weight.

She told us that she had times when was too tired to eat once she'd stopped for the night. I couldn't imagine that! I could never be too tired to eat!

Come to find out, our shuttle provider was a nurse. I asked her about breathing problems and high altitudes. I'd brought along two different types of inhalers for my self in case I got short on breath.

She told me that breathing should not be problem for us and that people who have problems breathing from altitude will encounter it at 6000 feet or more altitude.

Other than Mt. Washington, which is 6288 feet, we would be well below 6000 feet.

She explained to us what "trail magic" meant. Although we were paying for the shuttle, she was showing us trail magic with all the extras she was doing for us and explaining to us. I was so grateful for her help.

As we drove the long drive from the airport to Baxter State Park she offered that if we found out we needed to mail some of our things from Baxter she would be happy to help us. The park would allow us to that as we were south bounders. I again apologized that we would not be staying with her and told her not to inconvenience herself and just to drop us off outside Baxter and we'd hike in. She explained that this was a very large park and it was thirty-something miles into the park to get to where we'd be camping. She was very surprised when her cell phone rang because usually she didn't have any coverage. They were having unusually warm weather. It was in the mid eighties. I told her it was just as warm and warmer too in Florida. The heat wouldn't be a problem for us.

Driving in and seeing the beautiful mountains brought tears to my eyes. I felt as though I'd never seen mountains before in my life or, was I remembering back to when I had seen them before. I didn't know, but it was very emotional for me.

So she dropped us off right where we should be and we soon found the Park Ranger. We were told where to find our campsite and started hiking over to it. It was a short distance. Maybe a half a mile? I was struggling to carry my pack and additional bag and wondered how I'd do it.

We set up camp and scoped out the place. The bathroom was a composting toilet type. No running water here. The bathroom was newer looking and handicapped accessible having a grab bar by the toilet. I smelled the strong scent of pine on my way to the bathroom. It was like someone had hung up a car freshener, pine scented.

The Appalachian Trail starts (for a SOBO) at the top of Mt Katahdin and so, with out the resources to have ourselves air lifted to the top, we opted for the usual manner of hiking to the top. We knew that it would be rough but with brand new legs and borrowing a day pack from the Rangers station we figured that we would be alright. We had scouted out a little on the afternoon before to see how the trail looked. We determined it wouldn't be all that bad.

The day after our Mt. Katahdin hike I was very grateful that we'd had the foresight to book the campground for an extra night. I was virtually crippled. We'd come hiking down the mountain with our head lights on. As we were signing out on the register we found out that the ranger was about to start looking for us as it was 10pm. I was slower than an old lady coming back down the mountain. This kicked my butt. We'd started at 6am. Thank God we had brought along the Steripen as we needed more water than anticipated. The streams on the side of the mountain were so clean that most likely we would have been OK to drink it untreated. We never drank water untreated the whole trail.

For whatever reason, we ate only tuna fish from a can before starting. We carried more water than suggested by the ranger and we brought our Steripen with us to make more purified water as needed. Thank God, I brought the box of Cheese-its with me.

We were in a different world. No cell coverage. Miles away from anything. There certainly was not any pizza delivery here!

Every time I thought that we were getting close to the top I learned that we still had much farther to go. I was learning first hand what was the term "false peak". The sun was beaming down strongly. Although I'd been out in the sun some already at home in Florida, and had a bit of a tan, I was getting pink on my face and arms.

When we finally got to the top we stayed only maybe 15 minutes as I was very concerned, "how would we ever get back down"?

We met two women coming down the mountain as well. They'd taken a different trail up and were taking our way down. They had gotten lost the day before somewhere else and found themselves in tears.

They were greatly intimidated by the drops off the rocks. I explained that I was only watching the two feet around me and only sometimes I would glimpse a peek. They put on their rain gear at the thought of rain and were hiking around in their rain gear when they didn't need it. I thought about them breaking down and crying the day before and I thought that they were "silly and pathetic women". Sometimes they'd follow us while coming down around and over the rocks. I led the way for Rex and I. At one point Rex got ahead of me a little while trying to figure out the best way down. I thought he'd gone between two rocks and down. That wasn't the way. He'd gone around. As I came down between the rocks, all of a sudden I was out of trail. As I sat between two large boulders and looked down to the side of the mountain, I started to cry. Where would I go from here? If I had taken another step, I wouldn't be typing this today.

This was the first time that I learned to never mock other hikers!

We made our way to our tent and went to bed without dinner. *We were too tired to eat.* Thank God for the cheese-its. They'd kept us alive!

By the way, I learned that the handicapped grab bar in the bathroom must be to help the hikers on and off the pot. Yes, my legs hurt me that much!

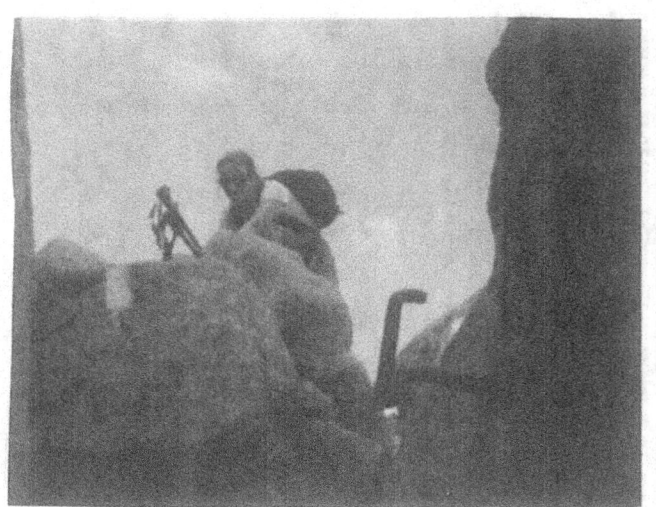
1st day on the trail

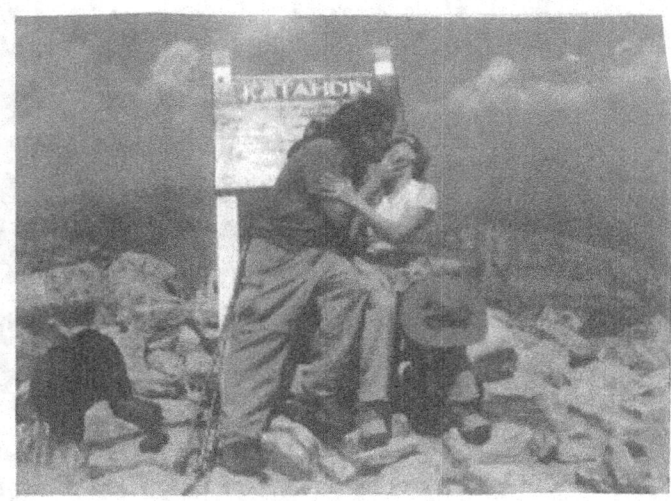
We made it up Mt. Katahdin.

WHAT IS THE PURPOSE OF THIS BOOK?

I want to <u>ENCOURAGE</u>.

I want for *everyone* to feel encouraged.

If you are not an athlete, If you ever feel depressed, If you don't get positive re-enforcement from those around you, or what ever your situation may be...
I want to encourage you.

One way that I know of, to help myself mentally and physically, is thru hiking. I encourage you to go outdoors and take a walk today. I don't care how far you walk...just do it.

There is no other way that I know of to get the same mental and physical health benefits as you get from a walk outdoors.

It seems that no matter how miserable I am when I start walking I find that after a while I become happy and prayerful. The sun on my face always feel good.

There's plenty of evidence as to the vitamin d effect from the sun and the serotonin levels go up as your body becomes more physical. You can not allow aches to stop you but you must be sensible.

You will be amazed at what you can accomplish if you give yourself a little moral boosting talk. Too often we talk ourselves down or we discourage ourselves.
Surround yourself by those that think positively. Don't accept any criticism that you don't deserve.

Always be grateful to God and ask him to guide you.

KATAHDIN

the first blog, from Monson, Maine

This is a good time for us to update this account. At this moment I have had a good nights sleep in a bed! My belly is full and I have on CLEAN clothes, and I showered less than 24 hours ago. Now I will tell you about the rest of the time...

We started off to climb Mount Katahdin by setting out early in the morning. We borrowed "day packs" from the park and used them to carry only what we needed; water and my extensive medical kit. A slow hiker does the climb in 10 to 12 hours. I won't tell you how long we took but we had on our head lamps to come back in. The mountain was beautiful, that is, what I dared to look at. For the most part I kept my head down and only watched my own two feet. Hiking around Florida did nothing to help prepare us!

The next day we scheduled ourselves for an extra day at Baxter State Park. This proved to be a smart move! We mailed home about 80 lbs of stuff that we would not want to be lugging around and set off for the ten miles out of the park. It nearly killed me and I had my first melt down. We were about to set out on "the hundred mile wilderness" and I was scared. Our packs still weighed too much and I was scared we'd run out of food, I was scared I 'd get hurt or Rex and could't get help, I was scared about everything. Well again, we lightened our packs and sent more home. We got more food and set off.

Well the "hundred mile wilderness" is not what I had expected. There was a very nice place to stop after thirty something miles where you could sleep if you wanted, get supplies and lunch or dinner. We took them up on lunch and some more Ramen noodle soup and set off again. (imagine, Rex had never had Ramen noodle soup before! amazes me) Well, there were not any school crossing guards or guard rails at the dangerous areas but there were plenty of people going by on the trail or going past. There are also logging roads that the trail goes over some of them are still being used. Most of my fears were unfounded. This has been extremely exhausting physically.

I am getting over the mental break downs. Our pack weights are finally down where they should be and we are "getting our legs". God bless Rex because he has never once given me the slightest bit of a hard time about being so slow etc. Now I am convinced I will not give myself (another) heart attack. We have been on top of the mountains and now I even look down! We like to stop and eat the wild blueberries and raspberries on top.

One day when I finally had gotten the hang of this 'climbing mountains' thing it decided to start raining. That really changes things! Slippery! Oh yea and then there is the first time we had to "ford" a river. We were tired from hiking and got to the river and I thought "oh boy"! "just like when I was a kid... lets jump the rocks". Well even though a rock is dry it can still be slippery even worse than the proverbial banana peel and I went jump jump and then whaaaaaah!!!!! I slipped and fell and me and my pack went half in, it felt refreshing but I was scared I'd loose half of my stuff. So, I got up on the rock with my knees bent and with the pack on and I couldn't get up for anything. The pack may as well have weighed a ton, so Rex had to come over and pick me up and help me across.

Then there was the night I got so exhausted and I broke down and cried when I realized we had 4 more miles to the next lean to so we "stealth camped" where we were. Rex did not sleep at all that night as we tented in a very small spot in the moss. But it was reassuring to me because he did not try and push me further and we stopped right when I said that I'd had enough. 4 miles does not sound like a lot but with a 42 pound pack on you and the trail is sooo difficult every step is difficult. One wrong step and you are hurt.

I have a new definition of R & R; rocks and roots! I am getting more confident in my own ability and have less anxiety about food supply etc. It is getting easier mentally and physically. Well, I am getting used to it some what but today my foot hurts. At first my legs were screaming at me, then they got quiet and my shoulders were screaming, then my knee, etc etc. As long as it keeps changing its OK ha ha.

We were coming out of the woods to the road where we could get to Monson and we are exhausted and we'd been carrying a ton of weight for about 12 days while trying to break in our legs. Our legs were getting broken in all right! And the trail goes over this little wooden bridge. I'd like to know what they were thinking when this bridge was being engineered.

It was sort of a rope bridge but it had wooden pieces to walk across. Only the wooden pieces were not planks like you might think but rather they were segmented pieces tied together.

The main side-rail section of the bridge was not solid either but also of segmented pieces. The bridge could bend any which way.

I approached the trail and I said out loud "you've got to be shitting me!". We were so close and not broken our necks yet this bridge really looked like it was a test. I didn't think about it for too much and I slowly made my way across. Rex, as usual behind me, was afraid I'd fall and get hurt and was perhaps a little too concerned about my well being and after I made my way onto firm ground and "AAAAAAAHHHHHH" yelled Rex as he fell over the side and landed down on top of rocks. There really wasn't a whole lot of water and Rex wondered why he hadn't just walked down into the brook instead of using the ill constructed bridge up above. Now I don't mean to sound so ungrateful to whomever installed that bridge. We-all do really appreciate it. Perhaps it was how tired we were and how badly our legs hurt but it wasn't easy for us.

It made for a valuable lesson though for us which is this; we should consider if the help being offered to us is worth it or not or if you are better off without it.

If a piece of rope is provided to help you get across a river should you use it? Well, we usually did but it always made me wonder if it would get replaced if it got worn too much.

The attempts at helping hikers along the way are generally genuine. With the exception of some trail blazes that have been removed by tearing off the bark on a tree or something of that nature.

The documentation inside the shelter's log book is usually honest. Sometimes it will have dirty things to say or in cartoon form and sometimes it is deeply spiritual and soul searching. I always enjoyed reading the ones by the lonesome male hiker who is coming to terms and working thru the things eating away at him. I hope that he finds peace thru God.

So here I am at "the landing" in Monson and we are planning the next 37 miles. I know it will be rough but I am not as concerned. We have met so many wonderful people! Don't ever assume any thing about anyone based on their appearance either. When we were on Mt Katahdin there was girl scout troop or some thing simular with the leader of the group being about 12 years old (or just looked it) wearing a ballet too- too! Then there was this real nice lady we met, slightly over weight, smoking cigarettes and wearing.... get this ... "crocks"!!! To hike tough rocky mountains! Well, she flew right by us.

I think they were mocking me! Of course I've gotten real good at pulling over to let others go past. But so far, there are a lot of people that have dropped off and also, thank you God, we have not gotten seriously hurt. Every day before we set out we ask God to watch over us and also to watch over all of you... our family and friends.

I'd read about pack weight placement and how men and women should carry the weight differently in order for the most comfort. I think it said something like...men should carry the weight up by their shoulders and women lower towards their legs. Or something like that. I never did fully understand it. But one day I packed myself to be a little heavier toward the top of my pack and I was trying to make it so that as I went forward up the trail and bent slightly forward the pack weight would push me forward. It seemed to be working for me. As I climbed up and leaned forward slightly I could almost feel a little push forward. "This is great" I thought. I went up another difficult spot and felt the little push as I leaned forward. And I went up another difficult area but this time I felt the push just prior to leaning forward. What the heck? I turned around and looked down and there was Rex pushing my pack up over his head. God Bless him but I nearly killed him. "I can do this myself!" I said feeling like a four year old.

REX GIVES BLOGGING A TRY

Rex' turn...

Well what can I say this has been an arduous journey. Something that I have wanted to do since my boyhood days. When I finally got to the top of Katahdin it brought tears to my eyes and to share that moment with my beautiful wife just makes it that much sweeter. Maine can be a most inhospitable place but not by its people. We have met some of the most wonderful people so far on our journey.

The first person that we be friend-ed was a man named Bob. He claimed to be a real slow hiker but continuously was ahead of us at every lean to. After we met Jack and his son Matt and his new friend Carter and they had Lucky Penny join their group. The four of them met up with us at different lean-tos and were a great moral boost for us. Later when the other three headed for home and we were all out of water at the next lean to (which was dry) Carter came strolling in and helped us greatly. I have witnessed first hand some of the most beautiful sights to behold. To go up mountain after mountain and to behold the sights brings you that much closer to God and his wonders. Nobody can imagine unless you were there how beautiful it is. To go over bald spots and see wild rasp-berries and blueberries for the taking was a psychological boost that was greatly needed. More later, got to turn over computer.

MORE OF COLLEEN'S BLOG FROM MONSON

So much has happened since my last update. I may get kicked off the computer at any time so here goes...

We landed at a hostel in Monson and was picked up by the owner. I was tired and I suspect a little grumpy and hungry and definitely needed a shower. She looked at me like a Red Cross worker would look at a disaster victim and she made eye contact with me and offered me a shower and clean clothes to borrow and a beer and anything else she thought might make me happy.

We made good friends there too. Two of which were Lodestone and Just Blue Skies. Sir Woodchuck and Boy Floyd were soo helpful. Rex's and my feet were killing us and we are nearly crippled. Sir Woodchuck looked at our boots and explained to us that the kind of hurt our feet had was due to the fact that our footwear did not have any shaft to keep our feet from bending and curling etc. Our feet are seriously swollen and I am wondering if this is a heart related thing. Rex's feet are just as swollen as mine and he's never had any heart problems. I ask other hikers and they say that yes we may get very swollen feet and ankles at times.

Perhaps also living in Florida we have less stress on our feet than people may have who live and work around the mountains.

We spent the day in Monson had some of the best bbq and made good friends with Tim the owner of Monson General Store. You can see the "house band" having fun in store on a Friday night. This totally did our hearts good. Just great people. Folk, Gospel, blues etc.

We of course went to the post office to send back home even more stuff we'd been carrying around. Amongst our things were two water proof boxes. We had used one of these for our electronics, head lights, cell phone and charger, extra batteries, and the other was for our medical kit. I hadn't wanted to give these up as they offered us protection from our items being crushed as well as being water proof. We knew that none of the hikers that had made it as far as Monson, ME would be stupid enough to carry the extra weight of the boxes. So we asked how much it would cost to mail them home. We had spent roughly $10. a piece for the boxes. It was going to cost about $10. to send them home. I asked "just for giggles, what do these weigh?", I was told "12oz"! WOW! We decided not to mail them home and asked the postal lady if she might have a boat or something and could perhaps make use of them. She took them. I think she was just being kind to us.

The next day thanks to Boy Floyd we drove into "the city" and got new boots. What a world of difference. We finally had the Hundred Mile Wilderness behind us and could move forward.

Next city stop was Caratunk. Caratunk was not what I had expected and proved to be just big enough to be picked up from and brought to a "real town". We tried our hand at hitchhiking. And I felt like a naughty teenager or a homeless person. There was a bus driving by and I thought "what the heck". Rex was real surprised when the bus came to a stop in front of us. The bus was empty excepting the driver and off we went to the next larger type town. It was a long ride and I was scared that we wouldn't be able to get a ride back to the trail.

When we were in the store getting our supplies I rather loudly mentioned that we were hoping for a ride back to the trail. The man that was a customer the same time as us said that he was in his work truck and couldn't give us a ride. So we went out to the road to try hitching back and along came the man again from the store. He was in his personal jeep now and he offered us a ride. We gratefully accepted. And with a beer between his knees... off we went.

We tent camped in the Northern Outdoors in The Forks. This is kind of a resort but also has a section for tent camping. For our $11. we also had privileges to the pool and hot tub etc. For some reason when I hung my blistered and disgusting looking feet into the hot tub the other guests one by one got out.

Then we set off with 50lbs of food hoping to make it past the next town and stop at the one after that. Well we nursed our feet as much as we could while moving forward the last real day of hiking was 12 miles or so over the mountains. It totally kicked our butts. Speaking of butts, I've fallen and broken mine twice. But truthfully, it was already cracked ha ha. So instead of hiking on past Stratton to go conquer more mountains we stopped and are eating big and resting our feet . Nothing but big mountains waiting for us.

There was a picture of Bob in the first batch of pictures. One of the first friends we made on the trail. He thought that he was a slow hiker but somehow he kept getting to the camp ahead of us.

We have met so many really cool people and Rex and I wanted to just move right in at Monson. The winters could never work for us though. It would have to be seasonal. It has been cold in the mountains. 38 degrees one night. Not kidding. More later.... Public computer library. Forgive all the typos.

God Bless and thanks to those who have signed the guest book here on line.

BACK ON THE LIBRARY COMPUTER

A typical day starts with Rex waking up (no alarm) about 4ish -4: 30. He is up making coffee and what ever breakfast is. He wakes me with a gentle "good morning sweetheart, here is some coffee" I take the hot cup and growl as I zip back up the tent. Then I sit with the hot coffee and can not fall back to sleep unless I burn myself and I think about all the reasons I shouldn't be doing this... there aren't a lot of women in my age bracket doing this... I've had a heart attack for crying out loud ... I've got high blood pressure, and not only that, I am right handed and have brown eyes! Some of my reasons are better than others. Eventually I begin to drink the coffee and just like a werewolf turning back into human form, I too become human again.

I can pack up everything except the tent from inside the sleeping bag. I put my clothes in the bag with me to pre-warm them. I fold up the sheet, handy to have, fold up the "z-lites" (thin cushion thingys to keep dampness away) change my clothes, put away the "head lites" (headband type things/ battery /lights for night use), put away clothes, get out medicines, ibuprofin, vitamins etc. then Rex comes in and packs up the sleeping bag. This is a major ordeal. Then we both take down and put away the tent.

We start off each day saying a prayer together before we leave the camp area. We pray that God will continue to watch over us and keep us from harm. We pray for good weather and that God will watch over all of you while we are gone. We start off on the trail. After ten minutes I have to take off my jacket. Another ten minutes and I need a drink. Then I have to pee and re-tighten my shoes. I suffer for about an hour until my legs warm up. Then I start to notice the beautiful things before me... mainly the fungus! (Well, I am looking down at my feet the whole time.) The mushrooms are so beautiful! I am not even kidding. I've asked Rex to take pictures for me. One looked just like a rose (see 1st photos) I've seen beautiful orange ones and the other day I saw purple ones. I've seen mushrooms that look like a sponge and one day when we were headed in to town and very hungry we saw a mushroom on a tree like a shelf and it looked just like a pancake with syrup. Yes, all of your thinking turns to food.

Sometimes I don't think that we will ever get to the top of the mountain we will hike forward and upward and I get so hot I think that I need to stop and then as we get on another side of the mountain and further up I feel cool air. We do eventually get to the top and it is so awesome and I thank God that I can climb up there and that my husband would want to do this trip and I am thankful that it is not raining. I've become such a grateful person! Rex and I will stop and pick some blueberries or rasp-berries and take pictures. Then down it is.

Often I'd think of those less fortunate physically who would enjoy hiking and for whatever reason can't do it any more.

Rex says that my size 6 1/2 shoes will be a size 4 double wide when we are done! I think he is right.

POST TRAIL INFO

I learned that taking my blood pressure medicine at night time worked better for me. When I took it in the morning I could feel it slowing down and I was causing my heart rate to go up at the same time. It didn't feel right. I also learned from a drug store blood pressure cuff that the amount of medicine that I needed had gone down. My blood pressure was very low and so I started breaking my pills in two. This seemed to help a great deal. I was no longer feeling faintish.

From the start at Mt Katahdin to the end of the 100 mile wilderness, about 14 days, my body weight dropped by a full 20 pounds.

MONSON, ME BLOG

There was a couple staying at the hostel the same time as us. I'll never forget the look on her face. They were a young couple and they were excited because as north bounders they were coming to the completion of the trail. They played out in the water.

When she walked by I noticed she had extremely hairy legs and a bikini wax had never been done on her body. I think that they were Portuguese. She totally didn't notice that the other people had noticed her appearance when she came into the store. The people at the store were all good people and they have seen hairy hikers before and they were not going to stare. I did not stare either but I was not used to seeing a woman with so much body hair!

She went about her business and had a genuine smile on her face the whole time. She had a beautiful smile that started from the inside out. Wow, she seemed so happy. I thought about how I'd been grumpy about not having any of my usually beauty implements. I thought about how Rex said that he prefers a more natural kind of beauty than the store bought kind. I could see why. This woman had a glow about her. She had a happy confidence about her. That is the kind of beauty that I want. Though Rex and I would both prefer less hairy!

Many of the Maine woman have different beauty regimes than those in the city. For one thing I think that there are more women in Maine who allow their hair to fully grey, often times keeping it fairly short. Leg shaving for women can be a little hit or miss.

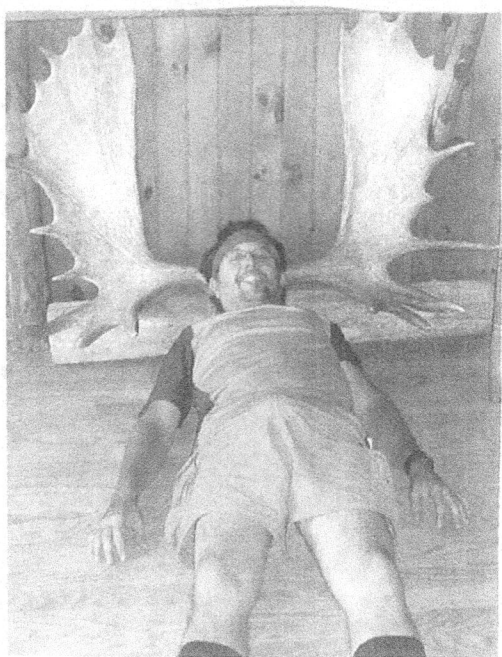

I hadn't seen a moose yet so Rex was trying to help out.

ANDOVER MAINE

REX and COLLEEN blogging

We have Finally made it out of MAINE!! The land of a thousand hands as I say, because they are grabbing at your feet and trying to make you fall as one of the pictures shows evidenced by my knees and arm.

We stopped in Andover, ME and took a zero day to lick our wounds and resupply for another 4 days or so to Gorham. Our trip on this stretch was very hard. Maine wouldn't let us leave with out totally exhausting us. This part of the trip we had to go thru the Mahoosic Notch which would have made Sir Edmund Hillary proud of us. The rocks were gigantic and only having on some a small toe hold to hold you with a 50 foot drop if you missed it. It took us 2 1/2 hours to go one mile which we were told as slow as we are... was very good. Most people have to take their packs of a bunch of time to get thru the rocks but we only had to take ours off once because we made a mistake and went the wrong way.

Colleen totally wigged out when we finally got out of the notch and would not go any further. Which I did not blame her because it was very intimidating even to me. When we saw this couple and they told us that we were totally out of the notch it was like somebody took one of those boulders off my head to say the least... it was very scarey.

The next day we tried to make a 10 mile journey to another lean to and didn't make it there until dark which when we got there we are totally exhausted. Hiking at night with a headlight on thru the mountains is something that you do not want to do. I think that I caught a touch of the flu from when we stayed in Andover because a woman hiker was sick in the next room. I tried to be cautious but to no avail. I am now feeling a lot better but had a rough night a few nights ago.

We have leaned that you can not make good time in the mountains when you are going vertically up and vertically down with balds that are soaked with algae and moss which made for a very slippery situation as evidenced by the picture of my knees and arm.... there was virtually nothing to hold onto but our walking sticks. Needless to say we slipped down on our butts many times to get down the mountain.

Sometimes there would be branches to hold onto but very little. I think that whoever made the trails in Maine had to be a sadist!

When we came across a sign that told about Mr. Avery and his donations to the trail and Colleen and I wanted to pee on it!

There is a beautiful library here in Andover. It was built in 1889 and looks as good today as it must have when it was just built. While we were in the library some boys came in to rent a video but the librarian said no because it was rated R and she would require Mom's permission. Also a young girl came in with her mom and was going to take out a book but the librarian advised the mom that it was from the adult section and contained "racy material". Wow! I thought those days were gone. Personally I loved it. I don't buy into the thinking that children should be exposed to all there is in the world. Yes, I am old fashioned in my thinking and believe that a child should have the few years of being a child to relax and grow without all of the burdens of reality. There is plenty of time for adult thinking and concerns as an adult. Do kids really need the complications of processing "racy or adult material". But that is just my thinking. Plenty of kids have full internet access these days.

The weather has been fine. It rained on us one night. But that is about it. We also made what we think was about a two mile error going on the wrong trail which Colleen wanted to kill me. If you have ever been hiking you know you don't want to go any more miles than you have to. The last 6 miles coming into Gorham, NH was just awful because I felt so bad. I thank God Colleen hasn't shown any signs of being ill.

Now we are looking to conquering "the Whites" in NH which Mt Washington is the highest peak on the trail. We will be above the tree lines for roughly 100 miles. So, we are a little apprehensive about the weather because it can get very severe and we have already been in some thirty something degree weather which to us Floridians is the dead of winter. But we have been blessed so far and I think God will make our way thru this. We still have too much weight so we ordered a lighter tent and lighter sleeping bags. I think that when we are done we will owe a million dollars ha ha. But it is something that we definitely had to do to make the trip easier. You ask hikers about going thru the whites and you get so many different answers. But the only way is to learn thru being there. Until next time .... hopefully we will have made it to our destination and we are looking for a level place to set up the tent.

We both go to the water source which is usually a small spring stream. We try to get water right out of "the faucet" I call it, where the water runs down.

MORE FROM COLLEEN

I usually do the "Steripening". A Steripen is our means of water purification. It is battery operated and is in the shape of a carrot. It works with the use of ultraviolet light that does not kill of the "bad bugs" but makes it so that they can not reproduce. Our back up method is chlorine type drops, Aqua-mire, they are mixed together in a little container and after a few minutes you put the drops in the water and you wait 15 or thirty minutes; I forget. Then, I usually help him out of his boots and into his water/camp shoes.

It is a small gesture that I make to show him how much I appreciate him and all he does and for putting up with me in the mornings! Rex sets about looking for a place to hang our bear bags. The bear bags are our food bags that are hung up in a tree with rope to keep the bears out of them. There are hardly any trees in Maine with good strong horizontal limbs that are about 12 feet off the ground and not touching other trees. Sounds easier than it is. He has however gotten quite good at "roping" a tree limb after many times. Then I will unpack the bags and set everything up while Rex makes our Raman noodle soup. This is one of the day's highlights for me.

Most nights are COLD and sometimes it has started to rain. He will come into the tent with a pot of hot soup and it heats up the whole tent. It warms my sore body and soul. No matter what time it is; it is bed time! If it is 4 o'clock we will take a nap before going to bed! I try to cover our boo-boos with antibiotic ointment before we fall asleep.

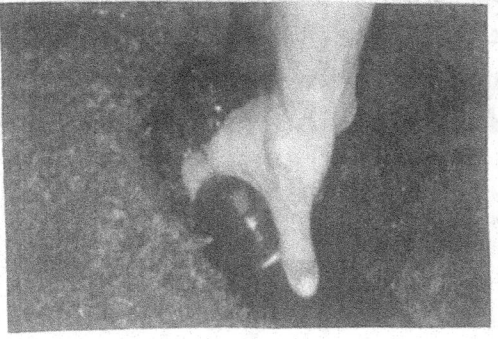

This water came straight out of a spring. Note the moss on the rock.

Soon we will need to do thorough tick checks. We have heard of so many hikers coming down with Lyme disease. We have had quite a few little spills. After a little fall I have all of the confidence of an old lady making her way across an icy driveway after having knee and hip surgery. Seriously... slow. I dig my hiking poles into the ground a foot or so and cautiously test each step. I imagine what I will do if I begin to loose my footing... I will tuck my shoulder under and roll just as you would from a moving car. I know that I would actually just land on my butt! So far neither of us has gotten seriously hurt. But one time Rex fell off a large rock and when he yelled and I turned to look at him all I could see was his face and his boots. His pack, rear end and legs were in a hole off the side of the rock. He had to take off his pack and crawl out and then retrieve his pack. It was not an easy day!

We will be in Gorham, NH next time I post..... that's right NEW HAMPSHIRE! There is a mile marker on the trail for the benefit of the north bounders letting them know that if they started back at Springer Mountain then they had just completed a full 2000 miles and only had 178 more miles to go. When we get to the "2000 miles more to go" mark on the trail we will celebrate having made it 178 miles and we will be going into NH as well! We will be out of Maine!

side note: When we got out of Baxter State Park (ten mile hike) to ABOL bridge we threw away some of the extras I'd been carrying. I had with me a bag of "Handi-Wipes' for when I couldn't shower. An entire stick of deodorant and package of disposable razors. And, I had hair dye in my supplies in case the stores didn't have my color! Where was I going to dye my hair?   In one of Maine's pristine springs?   Perhaps I didn't fully understand where I was going to be.

The terrain was so rock laden that to make yourself a little poop spot could be quite a challenge. While in dire straights one day, I thought well I'll just stick one of these rocks on top of it. It was a good plan except that someone else had already thought of it I discovered after picking up the rock.

CONTINUING FORWARD

We thought that we were going past the Jo-Mary campground on the trail. _I should have read our trail book more carefully._ The camp was actually 11 something miles away! A couple were driving by on a rarely used dirt logging road when they saw us struggling with our packs down the road. They gave us a ride. I cried as Rex and I again went thru our things and determined what we could do with out. The cam-corder was one of the things mailed home. We had two heavy duty umbrellas that we had purchased online. We'd read about some hikers that swore by them. For the most part, I just swore _at_ mine. The "heavy Duty" umbrellas flipped upwards when the wind blew. My eye shadow and mascara went in the box to be mailed as well as a large stag knife that Rex had given me along with pounds of other items as well got mailed back home. I determined that I didn't need to carry my own cell phone. We would get by with just Rex's. Some stuff we just threw away. We had a collection of yard waste heavy duty trash bags that weighed a ton and presented them as a gift to the owners.

Rex and I were just barely married. I couldn't let him see me like this; no makeup or anything! I'd hardly farted in front of him. (boy did that change!)

The kind owners of the campground gave a ride back onto the trail.

One day we had to get water from the next shelter. Not a problem I thought. It's less than a half a mile from the trail. I really had no idea how far that was but knew it could't be that much. When we got to the intersection of the trail we looked way down the rocky trail to where the water was. Oh well, we just took our time getting down safely. We ate our lunch and came back up the trail with the water we needed. We went further along the trail and all of a sudden the trail disappeared. Rex and I looked backwards and we could see the blazes. We were on the right path. Where did it go? After a moment of looking around my eyes went up toward the sky. Was that a blaze up there? I went a little ahead of Rex after I took off my pack. I'd climb up there and have a better look. Yes it did appear to be a white blaze. I went a little further on and there was another one. This isn't really the trail is it? This is crazy. I'm not a rock climber. I came back down and got my back pack. "It really does seem to be the trail" I told him.

As crazy as it seemed we both climbed up and continued on the Appalachian Trail.

Another afternoon we were making our way to a water source but there wasn't any water there when we got there. Oh no! What are we going to do? It took everything that I had in me to get this point. I will die if I have to go much further. Up the trail behind us came a younger hiker that we'd met. He was a college student who did sculling and he was carrying about 75 pounds (literally) and it wasn't really bothering him a whole lot. Well he came up on us and he could see by the distraught look on my face that we needed help. So, he dropped his pack and pulled out a waterproof sack pack that could hold about five gallons of water and he ran ahead and brought us all water. I know that we looked like a pathic "mom and dad, out on the trail" to him. We were grateful and felt it was safer when he stealth camped with us.

Rex and I were carrying so much weight. I just didn't know how I'd do it. This will get easier? I'd go by a rock on the side of the trail that was just the right height and I pull over and prop my pack on it for a moment. What a relief. We went by a waterfall where another couple had pulled over and taken off their packs to enjoy it and I thought "oh yeah, we need to stop here too" and as I pulled off my pack I swore I felt like I was floating for a minute.

AT A HOSTEL,
JUST PRIOR TO GOING THRU "THE WHITES"

So ... I always do updates after we have showered and eaten. I am much more upbeat! Here I sit at the public library looking like a homeless person. When you get to a hostel there is usually a box of clean clothes that you can pick thru to borrow while you wash your own. So, you try and find something that sort of fits or the all-handy scrubs attire. There is always another box that hikers can drop off or take what they want and need ; this is termed "a hiker box". Items like an Ace bandage, bug repellant, vitamins, sunscreen, are always in the box. Then there is always the zip-lock baggies with mystery food... is it oatmeal or something freeze dried?

Its a good thing that I left my engagement ring at home because it weighs more than nothing does and I might have dropped it in the hiker box ha ha.

We are shedding more weight both in our packs and on our bodies. We now have two new sleeping bags and a new tent. The "newlywed" double sleeping bag was great but extremely heavy. The new ones weigh in at 1 lb 10oz per bag. Much better than the 8 plus pounds we had been carrying. The tent was 7 plus pounds and is now down to 2 lbs plus a few ounces. This is very exiting news! Seriously I am almost giddy.

Your thinking greatly changes during an undertaking such as this. The other night Rex and I went out for dinner and I was looking at the sandals that the older gentleman was wearing next to me and I thought... "Those are kinda neat!.....I wonder how much they weigh?". I was never a slave to fashion but I have hit new lows!

I am feeling especially good right now because I was able to dye my hair last night!

I hope that you are enjoying the pictures.... they take forever to down load. They must be done individually. The program to bulk down load can not be put on these public computers. We bought a camera card to USB gadget at Walmart for the computers with out the card slot. I was big stuff yesterday walking around the "mart". I had not been in such an establishment in weeks. Nearly brought me to tears. ha ha

If you don't know what "the whites are", heres some hints: Mt. Washington is one of the white mountains and it is in New Hampshire. It is also one of the mountains that make up the Presidential Range which is also a part of the whites.

We are prepping ourselves for the upcoming "whites". We have heard so many different stories. Sometimes I get unnerved and find out that it really isn't so bad.... which is where the expression "hike your own hike" has come from.

So many factors play into whether you have a good hike or not. The weather is a big one for me. If it is not raining and a little cool .. I am very happy.

The whites have these huts that you can stay in. The AMC (American Mountain Club) wants around $100. per person to stay in one. No heat etc just basic shelter, a cot, bring your own sleeping bag and they feed you dinner and breakfast the next morning.

Many, many hikers try to do "work for stay" where it doesn't cost them anything. There are unfortunately a limited number of hikers that the huts can take with a work for stay arrangement. At the very least you can stop in and get leftover food, mainly soup, for $3. The fresh bread that the croo bakes is excellent!

About the hostel that we are staying at in Gorham... the main part of the house is beautiful from what I could see from standing in the doorway... all antiques and beautiful. Where the hikers stay is totally different. As you can see in the pictures. There are mattresses directly on the floor and beds were spread around upstairs in the barn. Privacy is non existent.

There is a church two doors down that lets you know what time it is... day or night. And, I know why the plumbing all drips. There is a train that comes thru a few times a night and the tracks are short distance from the building. If you have never seen the movie "My Cousin Vinny" rent it! The train blows it's whistle for about 20 miles before coming into the metropolis of Gorham.

Well, keep us in your prayers...til later

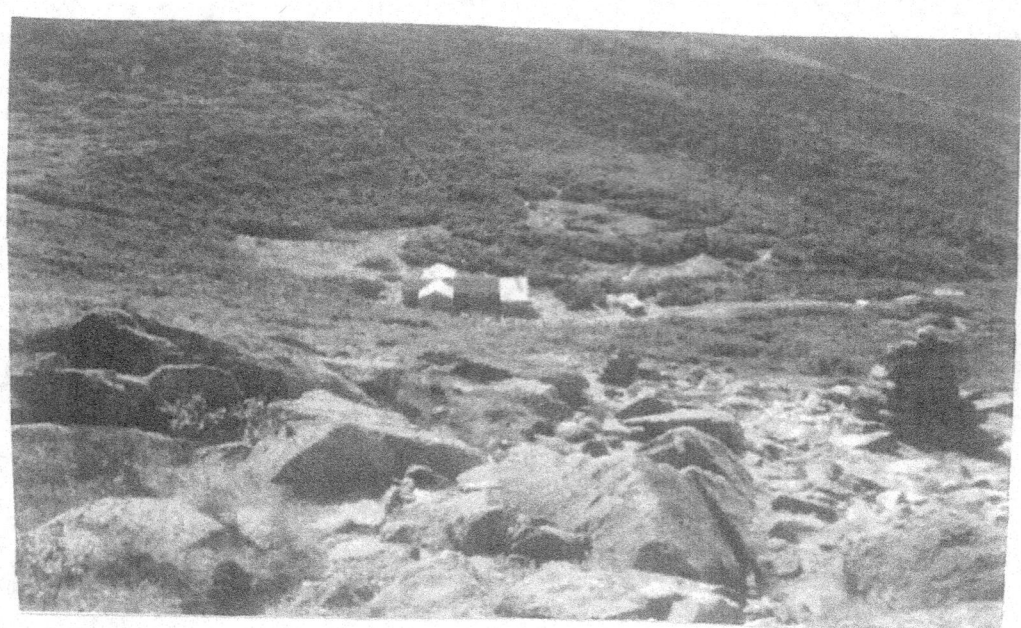

This is on our way down to the Madison Hut.

O.K. We are unable to download any pictures at this time...sorry. I will tell you what they are: a picture of a mountain, Rex in front of a mountain, me in front of a mountain. ha ha

When we last left you we had the "Mahoosic Notch" to look forward to. We again met up with fellow hiker Lodestone and the three of us stealth camped just prior to the notch. We would be fresh and ready for it in the morning. The Mahoosic Notch was particularly challenging for me. Everything that we have done up to this point involved using our hiking poles. These were new and confusing to me at first but I quickly learned how valuable they are and they have saved me many many times from serious harm. Well at "the notch" you put your sticks away and you must use your hands. This wigged me out emotionally and physically. I'd gotten used to using them to feel the ground ahead of me for its surety etc.

We made it thru the notch in about 2.5 hours. Not really a bad time. It was only about a mile but it was pure hell. I've heard of people taking anywhere from an 1.5 hours up to 5.5 hours. We were told to try and stay high on the rocks not to go down and climb over every individual rock. We did follow that advise but found ourselves in some very precarious predicaments. Having only a toe hold to get you across a long drop. Toward the end of the mile we met with another couple of hikers that informed us that we were nearly out the notch. It was a good thing because I'd had enough. When we got out I was so burned out and mentally exhausted and glad to be alive.

When we got to the nearby shelter I called a "Princess Day" and stopped for the remainder of the day.

Next we were heading toward some really big mountains.... Mt Washington and the like. Well we sat like a plane in a holding pattern and waited for the rain to pass at a shelter staying an extra day. There was no way we were going to attempt to climb Mt Washington on a bad weather day.

As we approached Mt Washington we saw the train go by us that goes up to the top of Mt Washington. I thought to myself "gee, we could have just ridden up there!".

It is an old tradition to drop your drawers and moon the train as it goes by. I was wearing so many layers of clothes and I had too much hiking ahead of me to participate in the tradition.

update:

While in Stratton, ME, Rex had his first mooseburger. UUMMM good moose! I don't know if it was really moose but Rex sure enjoyed it. We enjoyed a large lunch with Lodestone who was staying near by.

In Rangeley we stayed at a hostel. There was a young man there who went on to us about all that he'd been thru on the trail and he was talking big. He made us feel like we hadn't done anything yet.   Which according to mileage, we hadn't come far but we also knew that these miles were some of the most difficult.   He bragged and went on about all that he had been thru so far on the trail.

Later he also said that he was on prescription strength ibuprofin, 800 mils 4x per day. He'd had knee problems and had already had scopes and things done to his knees. He was carrying so much weight. He had a ton of food with him. His name was Please Cheese or something simular. He was stressing whether or not he could make it. We helped him go thru his pack and mailed ahead some of his food.   On his way out the door the next morning, I pulled him aside and said a short prayer with him. I pray he was able to complete the trail.

Just outside of Bethel, ME the trail came thru a parking area. There was a couple there, last years hikers, handing out chocolate milk and danish to those of us about to go up yet another large mountain. TRAIL MAGIC!   The calories seriously helped.   I literally felt energized after chomping down and psychologically it was a big boost.

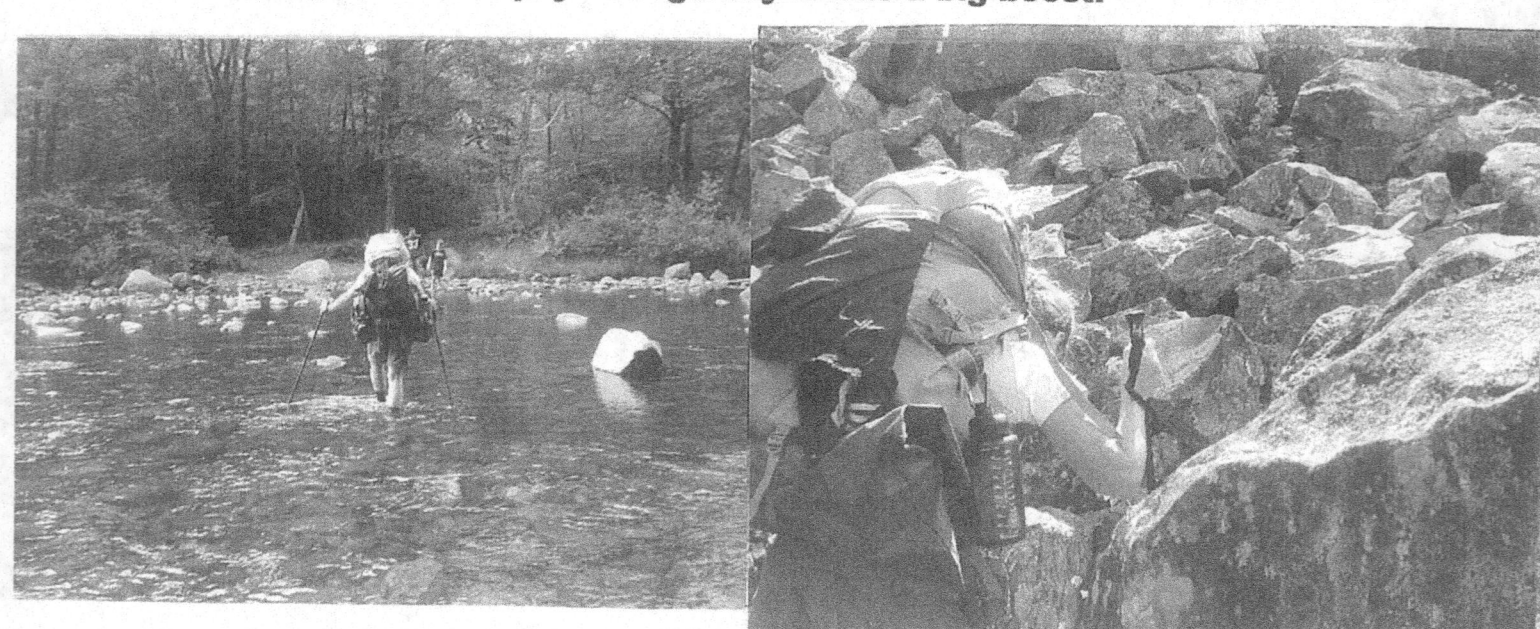

MORE BLOG

When coming down the mountains there were times that the trail would all of a sudden take a steep, steep turn. I would just look at the trail ahead of us and figure it would be OK we'd just have to take our time. And slowly we would make our way down the trail until if I looked back up I couldn't believe how far we'd come.

Sometimes a hiker would come past us and just bunny hop down the rocks as though it were nothing. Oh my God! How are they doing that? I wondered. But then I would recall one of the many stories we'd heard about so and so having broken their ankle.

One of the hostel owners told us that she had to get off the trail when she got a spiral fracture. I thought about the term "spiral fracture" and pictured in my mind what it meant. Yuck! how awful.

There was a woman that we met one day that had hiked the trail many times before. She told us that two years in a row she needed assistance getting down off a mountain. She was even air-lifted the last time when she twisted her ankle. I noticed that she was wearing the same sandals (that she had worn to hike these very rocky parts of trail) on this day and wondered if that was too smart.

The writer of one of our hiking books described his injury. A man's video that we watched tells of his injury. A woman we knew had a daughter that did the trail said that her daughter had to get off the trail for a period while she healed from her injury.

Sorry if we are slow, but seriously, we have lives outside of the AT. And while it does mean a great deal to us to complete the trail we will not do it at risk of ruining our health for the rest of our lives. We proceeded slowly. I knew that if we went slowly we could do it.

Sometimes it was a challenge to try and figure out which way you wanted to navigate through the rocks to either get up or down the mountain. Rex would often times go down the same way that I did. I gave him a hard time that I was testing the trail for him. I'd holler out if I came down on a rock and it moved on me. Or I'd say "this branch feels like its good" when grasping a branch along the side of the trail to help boost myself up.

CHAPTER 3
THE HUTS

We were on our way to start going thru the whites and stopped for a night at the Imp Shelter. There we used a tent platform. This was not our favorite way to tent camp but we obliged. There really wasn't anywhere to set up a tent because the terrain was so rocky and uneven.

It rained that whole night and again the next day. We were getting real acquainted with our new smaller tent. We spent the entire rainy day inside of our tent. Mostly we just snoozed off and on. I went over to check out the lean to just for something to do and found plenty of hiker gear hanging up and trying unsuccessfully to dry.

There was a caretaker for this shelter. It was a nice young man who wore a pair of women's flip flops that were held onto his feet using string. He told us about the ice cave that was there and how he could store food for himself. The shifts for the workers were something like ten days long. Much planning had to be made and if one ran out of something they would just have to make do.

There was an Ivy league school group who was camping there at the same time as we were. They spent the day singing classic songs such as "Singing in the Rain".

"Oh Boy!" I thought about how these kids would be our next world leaders.

We stayed at Carter Notch Hut (my favorite), Madison Hut, Lakes of the Clouds Hut, Mizpah Spring Hut, Zealand Hut, Galehead Hut, (skipped Greenleaf Hut) and Lakesome Lake Hut.

The American Mountain Club (AMC) owns these old structures up on top of the mountains. We were at Madison Hut the last year before it was greatly updated.

The weather on top of the mountains can be ferocious. We prayed that we would be two of the hikers selected to do work for stay at the huts. The huts don't have flushing toilets but rather composting toilets. They have spring fed faucets. Anything in the hut has to be carried up, literally, on someone's back. Any food that is not eaten has to be carried back down as not to attract bears. There are no televisions or computers. Cell phones don't work.

They have radio communication between the huts. If a hiker is rude at one hut you can be assured that the next hut will know about him before he arrives.

The young people working at the huts are amazing. Sometimes mistaken for "kids" working a summer job but the truth is they are anything but that.

When we were rained in at Carter Notch Hut we got to spend time with Emily who explained about all of the back woods training that the croo has. Many of the croo (proper spelling) have advanced degrees and emergency medical training. Rex and I witnessed first hand croo members caring for hikers coming in with knee injuries and hypothermia. The croo takes care of us medically, they cook for us, maintain the composting bathrooms, and carry all food etc on their backs up the mountains. All this with a smile.

The young women that we met were all well spoken and attractive. You would never picture them hauling 80 pounds up the mountain but that is what they do. They made the best homemade bread!

And so, anytime I'd here someone talk about the "kids" manning the huts I'd have to set them straight. Sometimes the croo would advise against hiking due to weather. If the hiker(s) went against the warning and got into trouble out there then a croo member would have to come to their aide.

This is truly sometimes an under appreciated job with out the respect due to them. Not so with Rex and I. We were silly grateful to stay in their care. Did I mention there's no heat?

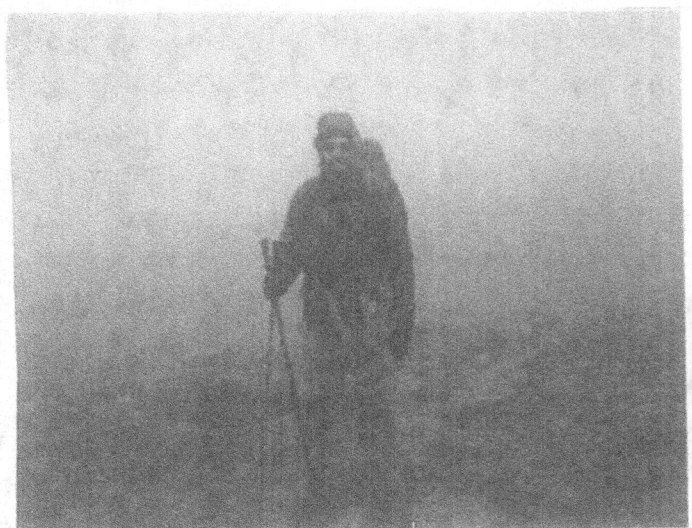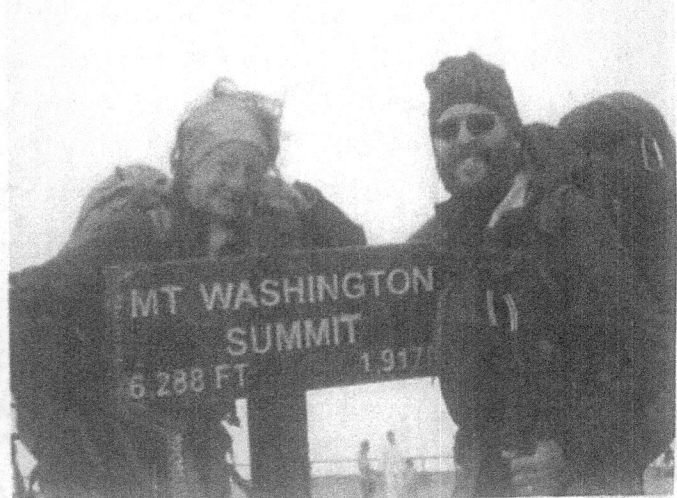

Rex as he is headed toward Mt Washigton from the Madison Hut.

31

HANOVER VERMONT

Here we are in Hanover, NH minutes away from VERMONT! What an exciting time we have had....We had heard such different things about "the Whites" none of them too good. After holding up for an extra day to wait out the rain we headed toward the first hut... Carter Notch Hut. Hikers say to get to a hut after 4pm for a better chance at getting a work for stay. (A work for stay is when you wash dishes or do any task asked of you in exchange for the honor of sleeping on the tables at night in the dining room and getting your portion of the leftovers from dinner and breakfast in the morning.) Sounds great to me!

Lakes of the Clouds is close by Mt Washington and is a really great place to spend a night rather than being out in the freezing cold. But the rumor is that the croo can get grumpy from being over worked from so many people and also there are so many hikers looking for a free meal that don't have the attitude that Rex and I have that is: that we are blessed to be in doors and eating a hot meal. There is a "dungeon" under the hut that is rumored to be awful and cold, less than clean, somewhat moldy etc.

So anyways we headed to the Carter Notch Hut with ideas that we could grovel, promise to work like slaves, fake injury if need be, or I could always work up a cry. And on our way to the hut another hiker had told us to ask for Michelle. So here we are up on this mountain and another hiker goes by us and I asked if she knew what mountains we were looking at and she said "why yes I do" and proceeded to tell us, then she asked where we were staying etc.

Well long story short, it was Michelle! We told her that we would shortly be at the hut begging for a work to stay and she thought that there may be an opening or two left. We got to the hut prepared to name drop and any of the other things previously mentioned and we were greeted by Justine. I meekly approached her and told her that if at all possible we would greatly appreciate an opportunity for work for stay. The alternative being outdoors with the wind whipping and cold or pay the $100. per person that any of the guests pay.

Have you aver seen the t.v. show "Touched by an Angel"? I swear there was back lighting above Justine's head when she said "sure come on in...we have room for you in the bunks tonight and some dishes that need to be done, we will give you dinner and breakfast in the morning".

I totally was taken off guard, I was floored. We were told to return in 20 minutes after finding ourselves a bunk and she would give us work to do.

So Rex and I found a bunk building with no others as of yet and went back for work. We were given a bunch of dishes to do and also some baking pans etc that need extra good scrubbing for the end of the season quality control type deal.   So we set about and we scrubbed and we scrubbed... one of Rex's cookie sheets was visibly thinner as he removed a years worth of brown and orange crud baked on the pans.

So, the croo ladies were so impressed by us that when I over heard them saying bad weather the next day I said "you could get a silly amount of work from us if you would let us stay another day". They looked at each other and said why not? Well, the first night we had other hikers at the bunk building with us...the second night Rex and I had a bunk building all to ourselves! We had our gear all over the place and we were airing out all of our clothes, we opened up and set up our tent to dry it, socks, sleeping bags everything spewed everywhere. We were dry! We were sleeping in bunks! We didn't have some other hikers next to us as in a hostel, snoring, we were being fed great!

One night they only had two paying guests and Rex and I We had beef tips in the most wonderfully marinated and spiced au jou and rice and corn on the cob and the most delicious homemade bread! A croo member came along with some left over peach cobbler and explained that we would be doing them a favor to eat it or else it would have to be carried back down the mountain. We died and went to heaven!

The next day we proceeded to climb the mountains called the Wildcats. It was not bad trail until we got to Pinkham notch which was a very steep decent.

When we were nearly down the mountain after about 2 hours of coming straight down we crossed paths with a NOBO who looked awful. Either he got drunk the night before or he was just not prepared for the climb and he asked us how much further. I didn't have the heart to tell him so I just said "you've got a bit to go yet". Then we checked on his water supply because it was dry for a long while for him.

We got to Pinkham notch visitor center with no place to stay before attempting Mt Madison so we stealth camped in forest across the road from visitor center. We were too cheap to pay the $65. for the motel/resort. We got up the next morning and we went to the visitor center to get a cup of coffee and a muffin. We should have just bought the all you can eat buffet for $10., but we were watching our pennies. We soon ate our muffins and drank our coffee. Then we decided to take a peek at the visitor center store.

Well, up to this point I had been using a rain poncho...suitable for a football game but not mountain climbing. I started to look at the gear in the store and I thought ..."wow! this stuff is great!". We purchased the best rain coats and we found a pair of rain pants for Rex and we both got light weight winter type shirts and other stuff as well. We spent $365. !

We went toward the rest rooms and we changed our clothes and we hung our old clothes over the side of the trash can incase there was someone worse off then us. We weighed our packs there at the visitors center after filling our water bottles. Mine weighed 24 lbs and Rex was a few pounds more. I was ecstatic! The difference in pack weights with the newer rain gear was noticeable.

Every hiker I criss-crossed I said "hey! give me five", as I raised a hand "I'm down to 24 lbs!". One NOBO that I remember in particular said "yea!" and he slapped me five and said "have some NOBO energy!".

We hiked up Mt Madison and stayed at the Madison Hut an dwe got a "work for stay". It was freezing cold on the way to the hut and I thought "gee, I can't wait to warm up!". When we arrived I again promised to be a slave for the croo and we were granted a work for stay and we were told that our "work for stay" would be to clean out the freezer outside in a small ancient building with very low (I'm only 5 foot 2) door ways. All I could think of was "perfect! oh well, I was already cold anyway".

That night the temp went down into the upper thirties and to say the least it was bitter cold for us. It was like a meat locker. We got the weather report the next morning and it said it was going to have 50 mile gusts and foggy but clearing before noon. So we proceeded to Mt Washington.

Along the way I was struggling to stick to the trail as the blazes were a little difficult to see in the mist and cold of the morning and I found a Blackberry camera phone. The phone had the owners name and information. Boy was he surprised to hear that we would return his phone to him. He offered to pay us a reward or at least for postage and we declined because we had been so blessed along the trail. This was our trail magic to him. He didn't understand the term of trail magic so we explained it to him. I'm so grateful that he could recover the pictures that he had taken.

We went to the top of Mt Washington which was so beautiful and we got the bowl of chile which was traditional to do. We proceeded from there to Lakes of the cloud hut about a mile and a half away from Mt Washington.

When we got there the croo had no work for stay spaces remaining. I kicked Colleen to start crying ha ha but the note from Emily from Carter Notch Hut got us in.

They have wind driven turbines for electricity at Lakes of the Clouds and they sound just like Nascar cars starting up. Needless to say, we had a fitful nights sleep but boy were we glad to be indoors! We left there and went to Mizpah Hut and got a work for stay there also. We stealth camped the next night.

I was getting so tired from hiking the day time hours and doing work for stay chores in the late day.

It is not easy for me to sleep in a room with a bunch of other hikers all of us on top of the dining room tables. We all went to bed early and got up extra early to be packed up and out of the way for the paying guests to have breakfast. We hikers would wait our turn and hope for plenty of left overs.

So the next day we hiked in to the next hut, Zealand Falls Hut, and hoped to do dishes in exchange for breakfast. The croo leader said "yea sure come eat we've got the dishes squared away". But I stood there and told him what good workers we were and we would do whatever he needed us to do.

Eventually, he got it thru my head that we could just eat with out doing any work. I almost couldn't take it. We were not moochers. We ate and were very grateful and we thanked him profusely.

Next was Galehead Hut who had a well water problem so there dishes were stacked to the ceiling. Colleen and I said "bring it on", for food, you bet.

One hiker that we met coming thru the whites also was doing a work for stay one night along with us. He said that he felt "degraded" by having to sit and wait our turn for dinner after the paying customers were served. I thought ...really? I'm just so grateful to be indoors and if I wanted to be equal with everyone else I'd reach into my plastic bag hiker wallet and pull out $100.

The next mountain to go over was Mt Lafayette which tore my feet up and I was a hurting puppy for a few days. We got into Lincoln NH and we took a zero day at a hostel which resembled the barracks from a war time prison camp. It was so hot in the hostel we didn't get much sleep.

We left there and now are here in Hanover NH home of Dartmouth College. The trail goes right through town. As we were coming down the mountain into town I could hear a football game in progress and I though "wow we are nearly there". It took forever as we went forward in great anticipation.

This place is awesome! We stopped and got a motel room. This is the first motel room we've gotten so far. I feel just a little guilty. Guess who we saw here? Our hiker friend Lodestone is here too!

When we were out getting our supplies a mailman told us to go to the pizza place for a free hiker slice of pizza. Free is free and free is for me and off we went for our free slices despite the fact the idea of pizza wasn't really all that appetizing to us. We asked if indeed we were to be granted a free slice and when we were told yes we ordered and decided that we'd split a drink.

We were yet again being cheap and besides we'd get something to eat at some other restaurant. The slices that we were given were so silly good. They had a brick oven and the taste was fabulous. We decided to stay. We'd order a large steak and cheese to split and also a large hamburger and onion pizza. We ate every bit of it. It was the bestest!

We only have about a mile and we will be in VT hurrrrrrrrrraaaaaaaaah. We are now increasing our miles. We did a 15 and a 17 mile day so far and we are hoping to increase that.

Some hikers say the whites were hard but I don't agree. Maine won that honor. Until next update we are well and are having the time of our lives especially being with my beautiful Colleen who has been such a trooper I am so proud of her I couldn't have picked such a great partner. God has blessed me. Bye

CHAPTER 4
MASSACHUSETTS!

It is Saturday night Oct. 2nd. We got picked up by my sister and brother in law. We are in Chelshire , Mass and we have been staying at their home in Ayer visiting with them and their two sons, James and Max and their standard poodle, Chloe.

It has been just wonderful visiting and seeing the kids. I have thoroughly enjoyed being in the middle of their daily lives. It has also provided excellent opportunity for Rex and I to get some things done.

Rick & Rayellen graciously lent us a car whenever we needed one. We have driven around and shopped for, and purchased, a new pack for Rex. He has lost so much weight that his old pack was no longer fitting him correctly and was causing him great discomfort.

As for the trail.... When we came out of the "whites" we came thru a meadow. I thought "WOW!" we have made it! We had level ground for a few moments. I nearly did cartwheels. We stopped and got some apples off a tree as we went by. Later as we came thru a town we were surprised to find out that we went directly by a deli/store and it had a small restaurant. Well, we had already eaten our oatmeal for breakfast so, we only ate one more breakfast each! We were so ecstatic by being out in the real world and all.

One day we hitched into town to get some resupply. As we were hiking in with our empty packs we picked a couple of apples to hold us over and I had to laugh at us. Here we were walking along like a couple of hobos, not knowing where we would sleep that night and eating apples found along the way.

Well, we DID find a really cool restaurant/store that sold Italian food. Boy did we eat! We left out of town with a baguette and a half pound of garlic and chive cheese.

Rex's lactose intolerance has been letting him off the hook on the trail. Normally any amount of cheese will make him violently ill but now, he's eating pizza and chunks of cheese etc.

All of the north bounders have crossed us and the remaining south bounders are real close by but at this point ahead of us. The trail is much quieter than it was earlier on.

When we started hiking in Vermont I looked at our book and thought "OK time to start cranking it up". Well, I guess I have to learn things the hard way because things don't happen in my time but in God's. First I got frustrated because although the trails were a great deal easier in Vermont than in Maine and New Hampshire, I still wasn't *running* up the mountains. Twice I can remember I got frustrated to tears wondering why all of this hadn't gotten a whole lot easier.

I am the leader of the two of us and I am to follow the "white blazes". Not the blue, not the maroon and yellow etc. So when we came to an intersection my eyes quickly sought out the white blazes, I knew we were going by an Inn where a fellow hiker was staying but we were going forward and getting some miles behind us. And so, we hiked along at a good pace and even had conversation! One thing that concerned me though was that the sign that declared the AT also declared "Long Trail North".

You see, the AT and the long trail both shared the same trail for a while. But why did it say "Long Trail NORTH". So I mentioned that to Rex and he said "well, in the whites we went north and then back around to the south". Well I did recall that happening and our guide book had told us that the two trails ran together for a period. Then we came up to a lean-to that our guide book had not told us about and I said "well it's a *bonus lean to*", "maybe it's too new?".

But it didn't look "that" new. So we decided to call our hiking friend. Fortunately we had cell phone coverage. Well, you guessed it. We were going the wrong way!

We hiked back and caught up with our friends Lodestone and Just Blue Skies (hours later) at the Inn and decided to stay as it was raining. We sat and had a beer and I was trying to figure out the moral of the story. All I could come up with was "don't be in such a hurry". I also had figured that we should be doing 15 to 20 miles a day. We have had a few 17 mile days but it is not the usual yet for us.

We had heard that Mt Graylock, the highest point in Mass., was extremely difficult. We met up with this husband and wife one morning as we went by a B & B and stopped in for breakfast. The other couple was getting off the trail. They told us about how'd they'd been told that the mountain that we were about to go up was the hardest on the whole trail. Seriously? I thought. We'd been thru quite a bit and no one ever told us this before. Was this true I wondered? Again I was getting intimidated. They were getting off the trail reluctantly. They listed off all the negatives on her health history and the list was very very long. I was amazed that they had gotten as far as they did.

Massachusetts was really one of the most beautiful sections of the trail and I had to wonder if it was the timing of the changing of the leaves or was it because I was born and raised in Massachusetts? This year was a bumper crop of acorns. Some of the trail had leveled off. It was steep for sure but it was much less rocky than ME and NH. It should be easier? right? Yes it was easier in that way but the acorns made it very tricky.

It took a little while but I adapted to having a little slide in my step. If my footing wasn't all that firm feeling under my feet I didn't fear any more, I would just allow my boot to slide into firmer position. And so we'd come down a steep mountain with our boots sliding into place while we tried to keep upright. It was a lot of work. I was frustrated. It should be easier. It looked easier. Sometimes my toes would hurt so bad from coming down mountains. I'd take a few steps then I'd turn my upper body to the left a couple more steps and to the right. I was trying not to wear my back and my knees out in any particular direction. Sometimes my knees would scream at me. My toes would hurt do bad that they'd stop hurting for a little bit but then when they started hurting again it would be even worse.

Then there was also the time that when our Steripen quit on us. I don't think I told you about that.....we were sitting in the woods messing with the batteries of our Steripen that wasn't working and eating lunch when another hiker came by and we started talking. Well he said he'd leave us some water at the parking area for us when we came through. When we came through and didn't see any we thought oh well I guess he forgot, whatever.

The next day we came thru another parking area and there on a bulletin board was a note with our names on it and a sales slip showing us that the batteries that he left for us were brand new and a gallon of water was underneath! We were blown away!

THINGS ARE NOT ALWAYS WHAT THEY SEEM....

When we first got into town we selected a hotel near the trail that had a restaurant and lounge attached to it. Well, we quickly found out the the restaurant was out of business. No problem there was a restaurant next door. Well the restaurant is closed on Mondays. Guess what day of the week it was! There was a restaurant a half mile down across the street... closed on Mondays. We went into an Eagles club....closed to non members. I was livid! There was a farm stand next door. Maybe eat apples for dinner?!

Lets look take a look. There was fresh bread! fresh cheese! baked goods! fancy sodas, crackers, yellow watermelon, beige rasp-berries, peaches and the best homemade ice-cream!

We stocked up and took it all back to the hotel. We had a feast. We ate fresh oatmeal/maple syrup bread, cheese and all that I've mentioned. The food was the best we'd ever had.

The room wasn't thoroughly cleaned as evidenced by all the kid toys and change I found under the dust ruffle area of the bed, the bath tub was not so good either and I wanted to go to the office and blast them a new one....but I didn't.

The next day as we were hitchhiking back into town a lady who was heading the other direction turned around picked us up and drove us to the hotel. She was a friend of the hotel owners. That was nice of her.

Then when I called the restaurant the next morning to see if they'd be open for business someone just said "yes" and hung up. Now I'd been hung up on! I wanted to blast them a new one! There wasn't anywhere else to go and so we went there and the waitress who had hung up on me was really nice. She was just kind of hyper.

The lady at the hotel was nice and told us we didn't have to hurry out the next morning.

Well, our Steripen wasn't working still and we had bought new batteries too so we got off the trail and bought a battery tester. Some of the batteries had been purchased at stores where the batteries most likely sat for a while and we were wondering if the batteries were any good or maybe they had been exposed to the extreme weather etc. The model that we purchased uses regular batteries. Another model uses special batteries that are more difficult to come by.

So, when the batteries tested OK we went to a hiker store with the hopes that the Steripen company might authorize a swap. Rex was so surprised when they said they would overnight one to us.

At this same time Rex had a tooth that was bothering him. He's had a couple of root canals and was afraid he was heading toward another one. Now we would take care of the problem of his tooth.

It woke him up at night and that concerned me so we took him to a dentist in town that we had heard about from a lady at the vegetable stand that I told you about.

Well, I had called Rex's regular dentist in Titusville and asked them to place a call at this other dentists so that they might know that Rex was a regular patient and not just some guy that hadn't been to a dentist in years. Dentists respond well to a call from a colleague's office (I worked for a dentist). Well, they were too busy and called over to the dentist on the corner for us.

We walked over to his office and left our phone number to be contacted when their electricity was back up and running (it had gone down) and we were walking down the street when a guy stopped his car and started to talk to Rex. He was asking him things like "I heard you're looking for a dentist. Is your tooth keeping you up at night?"

The bothered tooth had caused lack of sleep as I saw it on Rex's face. He didn't catch on right away that "this was the dentist!". He was seen later that day and the x-ray showed that he would be fine.

Rex was so grateful and sent the doctor a Case brand pocket knife and some chocolates for the kind ladies as a thank you when we'd gotten home.

Everything that I thought was awful and I should "blast someone a new one"; they turned out to be nice. It couldn't be that I was just overly tired and getting grumpy. Could it? We expected the Steripen company to give us a hard time ...they certainly didn't. We thought Rex's tooth would cost us a bunch of money, time off the trail and pain for him....it ended up being fine. I had thought we were in bad shape by being stuck at a motel with no restaurants nearby... the farm stand food was the best!

The motel people ended up being real nice, and finally the waitress real nice too. We were given rides to and from town by the nicest people.

One time a guy and his wife walked from their home to the gas station that we were at then later he came by in his truck just to give us a ride! It has been amazing how blessed we have been. Well, I am leaving you for now. As we hike I think about all that I have forgotten to write about and think about you all individually. All of the positive people we have met and the positive things in the Guest Book help to keep me going. This is the realization of a dream for Rex and <u>greatly needed therapy for me.</u>

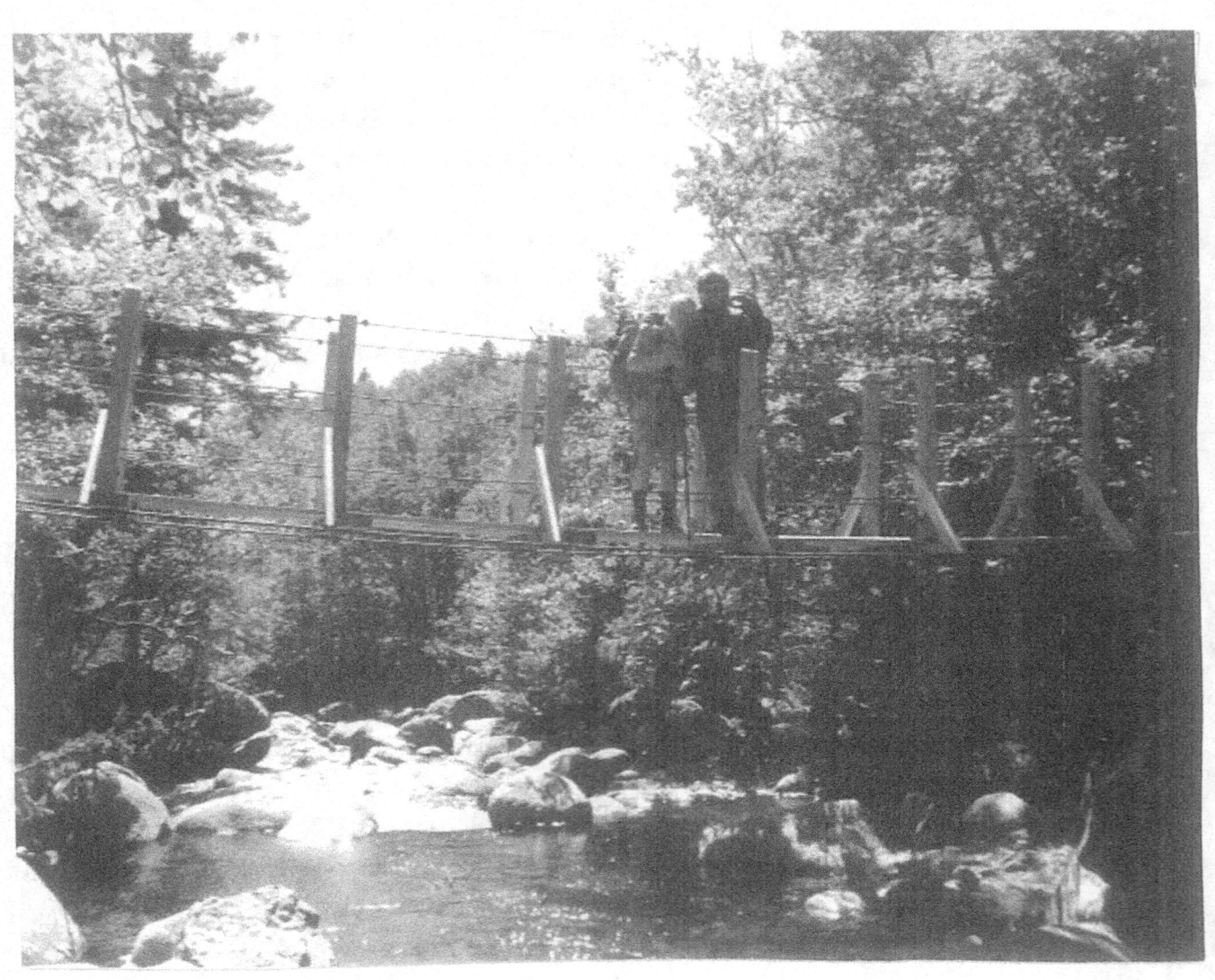

TOTALLY UNRELATED:

If you'd like to see other hikers on the trail what do you do?

I have a very strong bladder to the point that if I don't make myself go pee, eventually I will have a bladder infection. But even I have my limits. It seemed that anytime I would tell Rex to watch the trail for me because I had to go pee, the next thing I knew along would come a Boyscout troop or a church group.

So on this one particular day, needing to go pee, I observed no one around us and I only heard the tree loggers far away, so I began to drop my drawers when along came two people. These were not even hikers. They were two young people out on a date. The female part of the couple was all made up with her hair and makeup on. She was wearing high heals and was very self conscience. If I could have read her mind, it would have been saying "seriously, this is far enough, lets turn around". WHOOOOwA! Where did these two come from?

We went a short distance further and came out at a ski slope with a ski lift being directly in front of us. Apparently it wasn't loggers I was hearing but rather a tourist stop. I'm really glad now that my pants never made it down. Can you picture me with my butt hanging out while a ski lift is running over my head?

While we are on the subject of "going to the bathroom":

How *does* one poop in the woods? Quickly for one thing ha ha. I prefer to go to a tree that is not too old but is younger and has bark that will not easily break off. But not too young of a tree that will bend, because if you forget that it has rained recently you could be getting wet. I prefer to brace my self with my left hand, leaving my right for the dirty work. I will use the piece of tissue that I have stored between myself and my underwear, ready to go. I will replace the tissue before pulling up my pants. This helps to keep your underwear fresh.

I'll bet that is more information than you wanted!

BLOG SOME MORE!

I didn't tell you about "the Rocks" yet.......There was a mountain that we went over and part of it was called "the rocks". Well when we got to the top there were all of these cairns (little rock piles normally used to indicate direction or the top of a mountain, you can find your way if the trail is foggy). Take a look at the pictures I've posted. It was kind of eerie and kind of artsy at the same time.

When we came into the town of Chelshire we stayed at the St. Mary's church where they will let you use one of the two hiker rooms. We slept on the floor making use of the foam and pieces of carpet they had for hikers and seeing as how we were the only ones there, we could use all of it. I got such a good nights sleep.

It has been nice here at our families home having the run of the kitchen and I feel at home. It is surprising how I missed cooking! We have so enjoyed being a part of the family. We were only going to stay 2 nights. That would have given us one full day with them. Well, we had stuff we needed to do and we were having too much fun!

They took us with them to a Comedy Night Out to benefit the local police, to whom they had made a donation and were generously given 6 tickets for the show. As I looked down at the polyester sweat pants that I was wearing, that I had gotten out of a hiker box, and told Rayellen "these are my good pants!".

Another couple joined us and Rayellen asked the woman if I could borrow a pair of shoes because she had smaller sized feet as I do and so I wouldn't have to go in my flip flops. Well, this lady had feet like a Barbie Dolls and the shoe thing was not going to work for me. I told her that I had 6 1/2 s but realized after that perhaps I actually wore a larger size when wearing dress shoes not hiker boots!

I had to laugh at myself when I was trying to determine if flip flops were more formal looking when worn with or with out black socks. Then to complement the outfit, I had a "stuff sack" to use as my purse!

I was a little self conscience at first but what the heck, Rayellen offered her makeup to me so at least I had on a pair of eyebrows! I felt all dressed up with my eyebrows on and all and my hair was brushed too!

Lean-tos or shelters are mostly basic wooden structures where a hiker can spend the night inside or just stop by for lunch. They are used on a first come, first serve basis.

Having said that, it is custom for "thru hikers" to be given a place at a lean-to over a section hiker. Some thru hikers don't carry a tent so that they may travel as lightly and quickly as possible. Some section or weekend hikers will bring a tent along and only use it if there is not enough room at the shelter. Sometimes a hiker may set up their tent inside of the shelter if there aren't others around. This provides protection from the rain and wind.

Rex and I would do this at times because we weren't hiking "with the crowd" as most north bounders do. Our tent is free standing (does not require staking) and does not take up any more room than two sleeping bags. It also keeps the chipmunks from running across your face.

We would set up our tent inside the lean-to if we knew that it would rain and if there were no other hikers there. Even though the shelters are first come-first serve, we would move our tent if others arrived to allow them to use the shelter if they didn't have a tent with them.

Some shelters are a little on the yucky side. A shelter may have an overly used appearance (and smell). There is almost always some graffiti carved into the shelters. Usually there is a picnic table. Most shelters have live in rodents, mainly mice, sometimes snakes. Care must be used so that your pack doesn't get chewed on. Never store food or wrappers directly in your pack.

ALWAYS your food should be in a bear bag (some sort of nylon or other type of bag in which you keep all of your food) and this must be placed on a tree branch using rope. It is recommended to place the bear bag away from the trunk of the tree, on a branch approximately 12 feet from the ground. This can be a feat at times. Bear poles are available in the lower portion of the trail.

Below, see the pic of Rex putting our bear bag up. Note: a tent pad near by.

Some shelters are actually quite nice having an upstairs portion even!

Did you notice the electrical outlet at this one shelter? Someone has a great sense of humor!

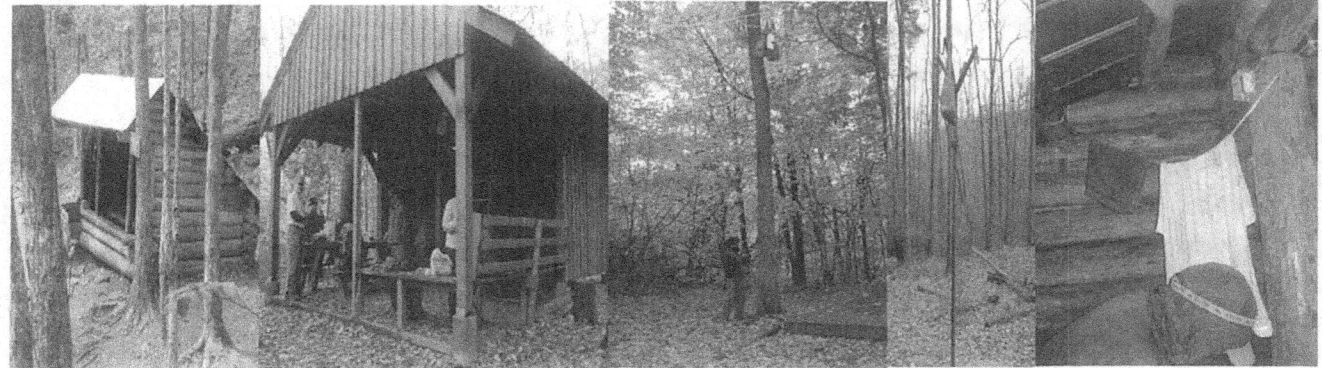

Enjoy the color pictures on the last page. The first picture is of a rainbow in Pennsylvania. The second picture is from Caledonia State Park. The third is one of our favorite pictures. This is the view from the shelter just south of Duncannon, Pa. It rained by the buckets that night. It had been raining for days. Everything was soo green!

CHURCH HOSTEL

Tonight I am sitting in St. Thomas's, a church in New Jersy, where in the downstairs they allow hikers to stay. This is a really great stop...there is a computer!!! a TV, refrige, stove and micro, shower and laundry facilities all open for usage. They might not be able to get rid of us! They request a modest $10. per person and share of chores.

It was raining last night with threats of thunderstorms, not the way I prefer to hike thru mountains. We were going to stay at the an Inn where they promised to pick us up at the trail head. Well, I need to read the guide book more closely because we were standing at the wrong road wondering where our ride was until we finally figured out that we had another 3 miles to go. It was approaching darkness, our legs were tired and it was going to start raining at any moment. We thought over our choices and I determined that I could make it to the next point.

And so, off we went hiking as fast as I could until it got dark and we pulled out our headlamps and rain gear. Well, we made it and we got picked up by the motel owner but did not want to leave this morning and it has been raining all day so we hiked over to this hostel. What a great place and we have it all to ourselves!

So much has happened since we left my families. I've got so much running thru my mind all the time that I want to blog and I can't remember what I've actually written and what I've just thought about writing.

We were heading toward CT and we stealth camped at night. A young couple, wet from the rain went by us and said they were going to do the "CT Challenge". This is when you go straight thru with out stopping. 52 miles. You've got to be kidding me.

We stopped in at Salisbury, CT and wanted a room. We were told at the only Inn in town that they wanted $330. for the weekday night. No wonder a hiker would want to hike right on past! We called a woman up from our guide book and she put us up for $50. She was a sweet 80 something year old lady and there were "no flies on her". She was quick as could be and loved the company that the hikers provided.

Rex's birthday was October 15th. Thank you to those of you who sent him an email or called. There's only so much to do for someone when you are hiking........ or is there?

Well we pushed ourselves to get into Wingdale, NY where I had read of an inexpensive motel that we could spend a couple of nights and there was a bbq place near by. We had already picked up Rex's birthday present at the post office in a prior town...what do you get a hiker?!!

A watch! But this is not just any old watch; this thing has an altimeter, barometer, it shows the ocean tides, moon phases, temperature, and with a separate attachment will make waffles. He loves it. Now when we are going over the mountains he can tell me how much further upward we have to go and if we have in deed reached the top or if we are on one of those ever famous false summits.

So, we went to Wingdale and got him some of the best bbq and sat at the motel. I must repeat. We got some of the very best bbq and the owner was generous and wanted us to be pleased. And we sure were. Rex still talks about it!

Well, when I'd first gotten to the motel I'd inquired about doing laundry. A lot of hotels have it available for their customers and of those that don't either have a Laundromat in town or because you are a hiker they will let you use the motel machines. Well they told me that they didn't have any laundry facilities and that I had to take the train to the next town to do our laundry. And I wasn't offered the use of their machines so I didn't ask to use them either. When we got into the room and I went to dry my hands on a towel, the towel felt like a loofah sponge...it was scratchy. No electric clothes dryer used here! What motel hang dries their laundry?! Well ....now I know.

So, we are sitting in this motel (also no phone, no soda machine, no ice machine etc) and I thought ..Hey! we are close to NYC lets see if my sister and husband want to come for a visit. I'll tell her that I'll show her all of the big sites in Wingdale, she ought to be impressed. (yea right) Well, when I called she offered us to go and stay with them. That was something that I hadn't really thought of. This was Rex's birthday and I wanted him to have full control over the TV remote and kick his feet up and eat all the bbq he could. Well, I hung up and then offered the idea to Rex; I didn't want to put him on the spot. Can you imagine? He wanted to go to NYC and visit instead of hanging out in Wingdale.

On his actual birthday the following morning we took the train in to Grand Central where we were picked up and with her handy rail card thing she escorted us around to her place. Then they said they'd take us out for dinner and mentioned a place that served "Pie -A- ahh". I'm not sure how thats spelled but it is something that Rex had a while back and wanted more of it. It's Spanish and made of rice and seafood and who knows what else. So the five of us including their son went out for piaah then we went to the movies to go see the movie <u>Secretariat</u>. Then we went back to their place for the most delicious carrot cake.   It could not have been more perfect.

Here I was thinking how Rex would want to watch TV etc and that visiting my sister was something for me, but no, he is all into his new family and wants to spend time with them and wants me to get to see them too.   It was a perfect day.

Where are they tonight?   Tonight we are at a Day's Inn in Lickdale, PA. Yes PA! So far we have gone thru Maine, New Hampshire, Vermont, Massachusetts, Connecticut, New York, New Jersey, Now PA. Next comes Maryland and then we start on the Virginia's. We will soon be going past the half way marker. I know what you are thinking... My God how long will this take them! Well, we are beginning to pick up some speed. In Maine and New Hampshire we only did 8 to 10 miles a day. Vermont and Massachusetts it was more like 12 - maybe 14.   PA has a really bad reputation for being rocky and ankle breaking. Well, it has been so much easier than anything else. We have finally done a couple of 20 mile days and one day we did 26.70 miles. Which I was very proud of. I think that the trick is that I am trying to get into town for a hostel or hotel. I am freezing my butt off! HA HA actually, we have had a couple of very cold nights and mornings.

One of my new favorite things to do is to set up our tent inside of the lean to. Usually the lean to s are full of other hikers but this time of the year they are basically up for grabs. So, we set up our tent inside the lean to which protects us further from wind, helps somewhat with warmth, and makes a convenient place for the rescuers to claim our bodies!

The other morning is was so cold.... "how cold was it?" you ask, when we took the top part of the tent off (the fly) and draped it over a picnic table so the condensation could dry in the wind while we folded the rest of it, well when we got back to attending to the fly it had frozen. I had to laugh as we shook the frozen condensation off of it. There are so many things I want to tell you.

There was this really cool couple that we met that gave us a bunch of food. We met up with them in New Hampshire when they were getting off the trail and they offered us their food. At first I was like..." no that's OK thanks", as I was thinking I was about to inherit someone else's broken up Ramen Noodles, but NO! They had these ziplock bags all labeled with really cool stuff. We got to try a great dry soup, chicken in a pouch, which is much better that tuna in a can.. more later, butter "buds", and a whole new to us kind of "Knorr's". Big excitement.

The other day we got into Unionville, NY and we were headed for a hostel listed in my hiker book and long story short this third hiker came to stay in the mini concrete block room with bunks and stay with us. It was a very cold night and we were all so happy to be in doors and grateful to the new restaurant/bar owner for making an exception as he is not keeping the hostel part of the business going. Rex and I helped the owners carry in the groceries and tried to look friendly and not smell. Anyway, Rex and I left our packs in the little room and went to the bar for food and a beer.

We were concerned thinking that she was probably going through our stuff and ripping us off as we had just heard a story about some bad hikers. When we got to talking with her we learned that she is a long time college professor and a very interesting person. She had just hiked 25 miles and showed up in town in shorts etc and looking a little worn. She was older than I had first pegged her to be and I liked everything about her. I'm hoping we can keep in touch. She really helped to encourage me. I told her that at that time I had not yet made over 18 miles and that was with tears. She told me that one day it will just "click" and I will go further.

Yes! I have heard the "click" and we have gone to 20 and past several times. Now I have new boots and I am going thru the pains that I did before of breaking them in. I bought the same exact boots as my last pair, online, a half size bigger and hoped that there would not be any breaking in period. But no, my heals are in real bad shape.

One thing that another hiker had told us was to get ankle support before going thru PA due to it's severe rockiness. So , before Rex and I left NJ we stopped at a pharmacy and bought knee and ankle supports. Then with our new bionic legs we set off to conquer PA.

A few days ago I said to Rex..."look at my finger" as I traced the outline of the mountains on the sky. My hand did not go waving up and down as in Maine and NH but it went evenly across the sky. I could have jumped for joy. And so...(unless I break my ankle) who cares about these rocks!

ANIMALS..... You are probably curious as to what types of animals we've seen... lately I've seen some deer quick stepping thru the forest and I saw one just the other morning. Later that day I saw two black bears! and two bob cats! and a porcupine and a river otter! O.K. .....the trail went thru a park in NY... (I just couldn't resist.)

THE FOLIAGE is so beautiful! The leaves keep me entertained as we hike for mile and miles. The individual leaves on the ground are just striking and I wonder how they became the colors that they are. Some of the leaves look like something changed in what goes thru the veins of the leaves. Other leaves seem to change their color directionally; either from the tip or bottom of the leave or perhaps from one side or another. Some leaves seem to change their color from the inside out and finally, some change from the outside in. Some leaves just turn all yellow or red. Now whats up with that?

As I am hiking along and observing the different ways that the leaves are changing color the colors themselves are dazzling me.

Sometimes I'll see an individual tree that is so magnificent that I'll say to Rex "just look at that tree showing off!".

My mood has been crazy, at times I feel like we've blown it when we are so cold at night and in the morning and then after that the temperature will be up into the 70s.

We have actually met up with other late thru hikers going south. Of course these are young people, from Alaska no less, that have lots of hiking experience and will probably finish in 2 months! But it is greatly encouraging non the less and our ETA has now changed from December "to sure hope to make it by end of Jan"!

I have no regrets though. Sure we could have hiked faster, we could have broken our necks too or not have enjoyed all that there is to see or all the great delis there are to stop at! (oooops) Now that we are more in with civilization we have discovered many great delis. A baguette and a block of cheese are our favorite things to leave town with.

Today was with mixed emotion. We stopped in to the town, Vernon, NJ , and there was a giant A & P. It had everything you could ever want including a wide selection of fresh baked goods. Well, tomorrow we go thru another town with some sort of grocery store and another not too far after that. I hate carrying food and I was really grumpy last town when we left carrying food enough for 4 to 5 days. The smallest amount of weight feels like a ton to carry it all day. To not carry enough and be with out snack food is also miserable. It is a difficult balance to carry just what is needed, not too much, have enough to actually eat well, not to run out etc..

I am very tired and want to join Rex on the little sofa to watch TV. more later, I will be thinking about all of you on the trail...God Bless

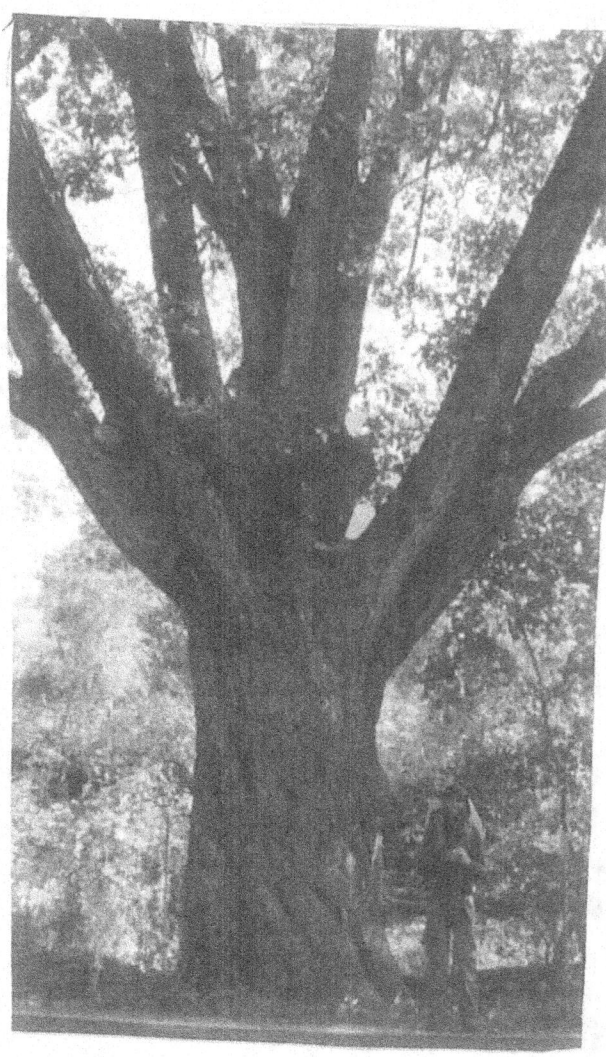

Largest Oak Tree on A.T.
Dover Oak
20 feet 4 inches

Its the climbs and the descents that kill me! Sometimes when we are coming down a mountain and switch backing ..back and forth.. I feel like I am in a European Army with my toes pointing and coming straight down heavily. Or sometimes I feel like I've been stuck in a game of Super Mario Brothers, going back and forth up and down. Sometimes when we are coming down into a gap the trail will go around and down and around like one of those wishing well things that you drop a coin into and watch it go around and around and down. My toes scream at me after a while and the pads of my feet ache. We have been having fun in PA so far. Unless there is something really huge coming up for us that I can't even fathom; this is way easier than anything else. I can't wait for Maryland and the Virginia's are supposed to be nice trail. I won't even know how to act.

We stayed at another church hostel the other night. The woman Reverend came out and talked with us hikers. She was very nice and I enjoyed talking to her.

I didn't even tell you about the Monastery that we stayed at in NY. It got late and I was bout to say "lets just set up our tent in the middle of the trail!" as we pulled on our head lamps. There was supposed to be a monastery basically in the middle of the woods. I didn't see any neon signs that said "this way to monastery" and I had visions of monks that didn't speak and stomped on grapes etc and then we came across it. WOW what a large facility. Those Catholics don't fool around. There was a pavilion in the ball field that was available to us hikers. It had an outdoor shower, port o lets, electricity and lights! We were ecstatic. We could recharge the cell phone and have lights on while we set up our tent under the pavilion. And not to mention in the morning I could curl my hair. O.K. actually I had to ditch the curling iron. (just making sure that you are still paying attention)

We stayed at the Mohican Outdoor Center, just off the trail, in NY. I loved it. There were these very large cabins with individual rooms and lots of bathrooms, and a refrigerator and full cooking facilities. If it had a TV we would still be there. Our room came with a separate electric heater in addition to the thermostat on the wall. I cranked up the heat and had it blasting in our room. We were sleeping in our skivvies and it was freezing outside.

When we went into town one time for resupply and showers we stayed at this hotel that was so dirty. You know, its one thing to be in your own dirt but 'who knows who's dirt' is something else. That's one of the things normally about staying in the hostels, they can be crowded with smelly people (fellow hikers). This time of the year we either have the place all to ourselves or perhaps share it with one other hiker.

When we stay in doors I have a little routine. First I open up the tent and spread it out to dry the condensation, rain etc. Then I set about washing socks and underwear in the sink. I take the socks and put them over the handles of our hiking poles to dry and set them near a heat source or I'll set up a fan for faster drying. You can only imagine how great the room smells by now!

One hotel we stayed at did not have laundry facilities so I did my sink laundry and set up the hair dryer to stand up using a spare roll of toilet paper and aimed it at the towel rack where our socks and undies hung.

Here's a good one; one day we did 26.70 miles so that we could land in town and stay at a cheap hotel that I'd read about. When its cold out I guess I find new energy! We were headed into Port Clinton and when we hiked toward the lights (it was getting dark) I was so excited we had done it. I slapped Rex a high five because I had anticipated that we would be in the hotel in about 45 minutes. It was really hard but we had made good time. Sometimes as you are headed into town it will look like you are going past the town and then you will turn and head directly into town. So when it appeared that we were headed away from the town, I thought, "it'll turn back again", but no. This time we kept going and I just didn't understand but of course we stayed on the trail and we came out on a road where there was construction being done on an overpass.

We hiked around down the street because I figured there was some reason why the grass had been cut. We couldn't find the trail anywhere. How could it just disappear? We finally asked a couple of guys parked in a car and they pointed down the road in the opposite direction.

So again we hiked off. Now I was getting excited because I remembered a couple of the business names that I was seeing from inside the hiker guide. Yippee! We finally did it! We hiked the entire 26.7 miles and now we would go to the hotel and have a burger and a beer in the restaurant there! I was so excited and proud of us. Of course my feet understandably were real sore. It was also very very cold. Stopping to look around and find the trail really let me know how cold it was and so we hiked into Port Clinton, and we went right up to the hotel.

Wouldn't you know it! The hotel is closed on Mondays and YOU KNOW what day of the week it was. Here I was, so tired, my feet wouldn't even talk to me anymore. It was freezing cold and dark out. I could hear music playing inside where the innkeeper stayed. I nearly pounded down the door. Some poor nice young man made the mistake of jogging past when I nearly grabbed him and said pathetically "will you help us!". What a nice young man he was and he drove us to a hotel in the next town. We offered him some gas money for his short trip and thanked him profusely. He refused any money though because he said that he had been in some bad situations and people have helped him and he was just paying it forward.

There were all kinds of cool businesses there too. The next day Rex and I spent HOURS at the huge outfitters. They have a cafe and we nearly moved in. We left with new socks and a few other cool things. Mostly we would find something that we thought was neat and then weighing it in our hands we'd say "naaaah".

Speaking of moving in; this hotel is great! It is $50. clean etc. We have our own microwave, refrigerator, computer usage in the foyer, and I'm thinking... if they will allow cats here then Rex and I should seriously consider moving in. Imagine, the heat/ AC is included, endless hot water, free continental breakfast, cable TV, clean towels and sheets, Internet. What a bargain. That is $1400. a month.

Currently Rex is upstairs waiting for his Gators game to come on. But don't think that it is all easy. Tomorrow night I will be back on hard ground sleeping in the tent.

Tomorrow we will be hiking and I will be thinking about all that I did not yet tell you... like how in NH when we came hiking in at night with our headlights on how pretty the rocks looked with all of the mica sparkling or how a month later when coming in at night how the leaves looked absolutely neon, bright colors.

PS new pictures to follow later

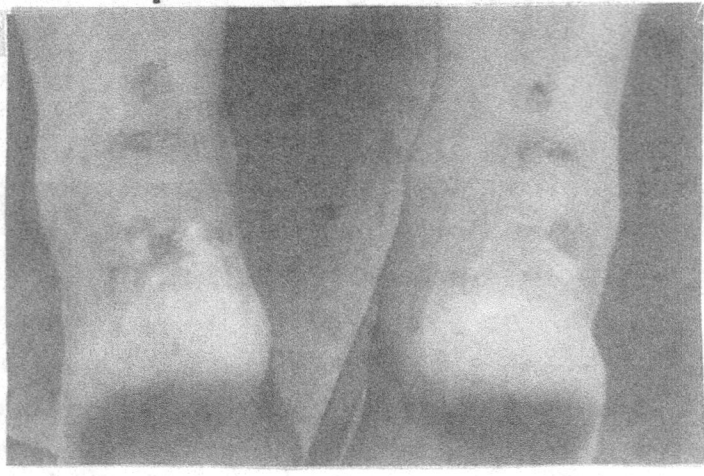

Colleen's oozing blisters on her heals.

Duncannon is one a place that hikers often discuss. The trail goes straight thru this town and we'd heard so many stories about The Doyle Hotel. We came hiking down the mountain over the railroad tracks and out to a highway. Our book showed only one set of railroad tracks when actually there were two different sets of tracks on different ends of town. This set us about going down a highway the wrong way. There were faint white blazes so we thought that we were going the right way. The traffic went by quickly.

We hiked past a memorial to a woman that had died at this scene. Really! make me hike past where someone else got killed. We ran out of white blazes and had to turn around and eventually we went in the right direction.

We stopped in at The Doyle Hotel and had the best steak. I usually won't pay for steak and I don't often crave one but somehow I knew that it would be good. We found the owners to be great people and we could see why so many hikers had told us about them.

We placed an order by phone to get us some warmer gloves and they were going to arrive in two days. When we went to pick them up at the post office they weren't there. We called the company and were told that the post office turned away the package? What! We'd had items shipped to other post offices and they were received. I'd called ahead to a couple of post offices to make sure that they would accept a delivery from another shipper and I was told it wasn't a problem.

Well, whoever was the postmaster at this location said that it was against post office regulations. Oh great! We had the package resent thru the U.S.P.S. to the post office. This cost us more time and of course more money.

CHAPTER 5

HALF WAY!

We've gone past the AT midpoint. Finally!

We stopped in Caledonia Park and tent camped for the night. There were coin operated showers there. So we got some change and went in. It was very cold out but the showers were nice and warm. So Rex and I shared one for about $15. worth!   I calculated what it would cost to spend the night with the shower on. This somehow seemed reasonable to me, and it came out to roughly $40.. "That's not really all that bad" I thought. I knew that we'd look like raisins though.   God I love these tank-less water heaters.

We opted for slepping in the tent instead and wiped ourselves off with our hands as we didn't have any towels.

We stopped in a bar because I had called ahead and was assured that they had food there. Yes they had food, but we had no money! We sat at the bar drinking our coffees and decided on tuna fish sandwiches for the next days lunch.   We would have just enough money for this. We struck up conversation with a man there and when we went to pay the barmaid we were told that he had picked up our tab. We could not be more thankful.

Much later we tracked down an address for him and we sent him a thank you note and Rex included a Case brand pocket knife.

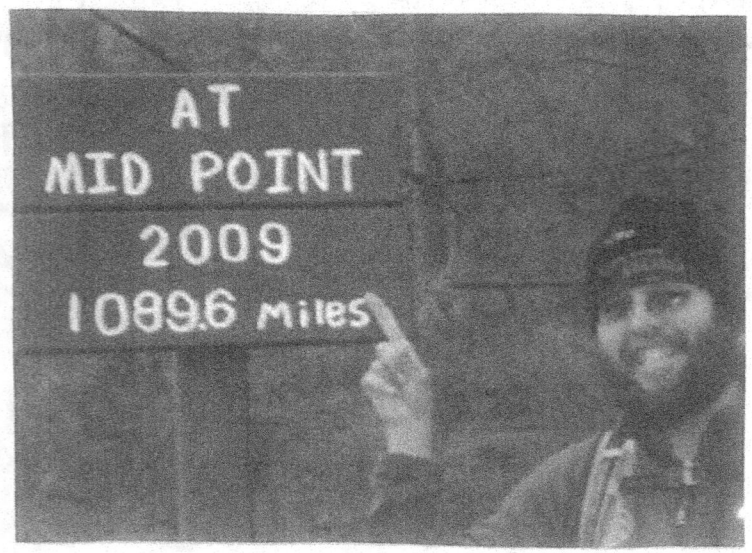

Guess, "where's Rex?"

56

Harpers Ferry!!

This town is even more talked about than Duncannon. It is the location of the Appalachian Trail Conservancy. Everyone wants to make it to this point. Although it is not really the half way mark it is considered to be.

This is a historical town. It is the place where The John Brown Harpers Ferry Raid took place prior to the Civil War. This place is silly with history and the buildings and homes are really cool. It was beautiful to look up at Harpers Ferry and see its streets. There were steps up from one street to another. We stayed at a historical inn. It was great but no TV. The owner was adamant about no TV. I understood our need to interact with one another but did she fully understand what it was like to be a hiker?

The majority of hikers go solo and the only form of entertainment came from their interactions with other hikers. (A few hikers had headsets for music/radio.) As a hiker you always are looking for weather information. Although getting away from society is one of the greatest parts of hiking you do sometimes want to know what is going on in the world.

The B.P. oil spill happened during our hike. I couldn't believe how long it took to stop it.

When we left Harpers Ferry we were hiking up yet another mountain and we got to see groups of deer right along the path. It was beautiful to see the deer with the mountains for a backdrop. This is one of the reasons for doing the trail. Some of the things that we have seen seem make believe.

The Bear's Den!

This hostel was really neat and historical. We were so grateful to have a warm place to spend the night and we enjoyed talking to the volunteer couple staying there. Of course the pizza and all that could be purchased were also warmly received.

FRONT ROYAL (1st time)

We had a great Thanksgiving stopping in on the most wonderful bed and breakfast; Burgundy Lane B & B in Waynesboro, PA. I'd seen an advertisement and thought I'd call just for giggles and find out how much it cost. I felt certain that it would be too much money. I was surprised when I learned how reasonable it would be. I asked the owners twice, "now this is for two, right?".

Dave came out and got us and even stopped by the local mart so I could pick up contact lenses. The next morning we had the best breakfast. I'd love to go back there.

It is Tues. Dec.7th and we are at a hotel in Front Royal, VA. Now, we are about to head out into the Shenandoah and I'm not sure how this will go for us. It is getting pretty darned cold! We have only had a sprinkling of snow but the wind! We have purchased some of those hand warming things and I plan to use some for my feet at bedtime. We set up the tent in a lean to at night to cut back on the amount of wind and we make it a short day. The inside of the tent gets to a manageable temperature using our sleeping bags, liners, and nearly all of the clothing that we carry. I have a couple of times put my rain pants on over my clothes for additional warmth. Going pee is awful!

Rex usually makes soup or something hot for us after we get the tent set up. This helps greatly with heating up the tent and sure makes you feel good to have some warm soup. The inside of the tent gets covered with condensation and is always wet. When we get out in the morning the tent freezes and so we shake off the water before rolling it up. We have thought about and talked about stopping and resuming in April. Sometimes I fantasize about coming home for the holidays... hot chocolate, hot baths ... warm warm warm. If we do stop for a while it will be o.k.. But, part of me will feel defeated because it has not been part of our plan. Perhaps I need to cut myself a break? If I can say .."I finished last", it will only be the first two words that count.

I imagine restarting in April breaking back in my trail legs. There are many benefits to being "late in the season" hikers. The lean-tos are almost always ours solely. There are less chances of Lyme Disease, less mosquitos, the hostels (those that are open) are all ours, the hotels give you better off season rates and when out on the trail you can pee where and when you feel the need! We will go forward until it becomes to silly to go further. Who knows, maybe we can do it in one try.

If we complete the whole trail in one years time we will be considered "thru hikers" which has been one of our goals. We have not cheated in any way. Many hikers skip parts of the trail. We have also not "slack packed"; having someone drive your pack ahead for you, which this is not cheating but it was not how Rex had defined our hike. Just about every time I think its time to stop and get off the trail, we have a really great day. Sometimes it is someone that we meet, sometimes it is where we are hiking. We have been on an adventure and it has been great We have come thru some crazy historical places and seen some really cool things.

If we can hang in there for another week or two we will be much further south and the weather warmer. When we don't have good days anymore we will put it down like an old dog with mixed emotions. These old dogs WILL finish one way or another though. This trip has allowed me to become more relaxed than I ever have been. It has also reawakened parts of me that I thought were nearly dead.

This time that Rex and I have shared could not be bought. We have both been blessed in some many ways. When we decided to get married I was using the smart part of my brain, the part that guided me out of the bad situation I had been in prior and while I knew that us getting married was the right thing to do...(part of me was still guarded), I feel more confident in our relationship now. We have gotten much closer and I have no doubts that God has brought us together.

One day we were hiking along and I stopped and turned to Rex with tears rolling down my face and I said "I get it !". People do the AT for many reasons, some don't know why they just feel a need to do it. The answer for me wasn't really an epiphany, it just became clear. It is a feeling that most of us haven't felt it since we were kids:those of us who were blessed to have decent childhoods have felt it. It is a comfort. It is knowing that we are o.k., that we are loved by God and there is an absence of worry. There is a confidence that I can only describe like this; when I was small and my mom bought me a new pair of sneakers I just knew that I could run faster now!

There isn't enough Zoloft in the world to make you feel this good and I have felt it. I continue to feel it. This trail has been my therapy for sure.

Never in my adult life have I been at a better place in my life. I am with a man, my husband, who truly loves me. We have a nice home to go to and unless we really go crazy and stupid, we can afford it. I have health insurance and a car that I have the title to; no payments. Granted its a 1998 but it is all mine! (ours)

My daughter is grown now and while I know that I have made mistakes in the ways that I raised her, I always tried my best and I prayed the whole time for her well being. Now I can do no more for her except to be on the side lines and to be her cheer leader just as my dad has done for me.

About those hand warming things; I learned that if I placed them in my upper leg/crotch area, where there is a main artery, I had a feeling of being warm.

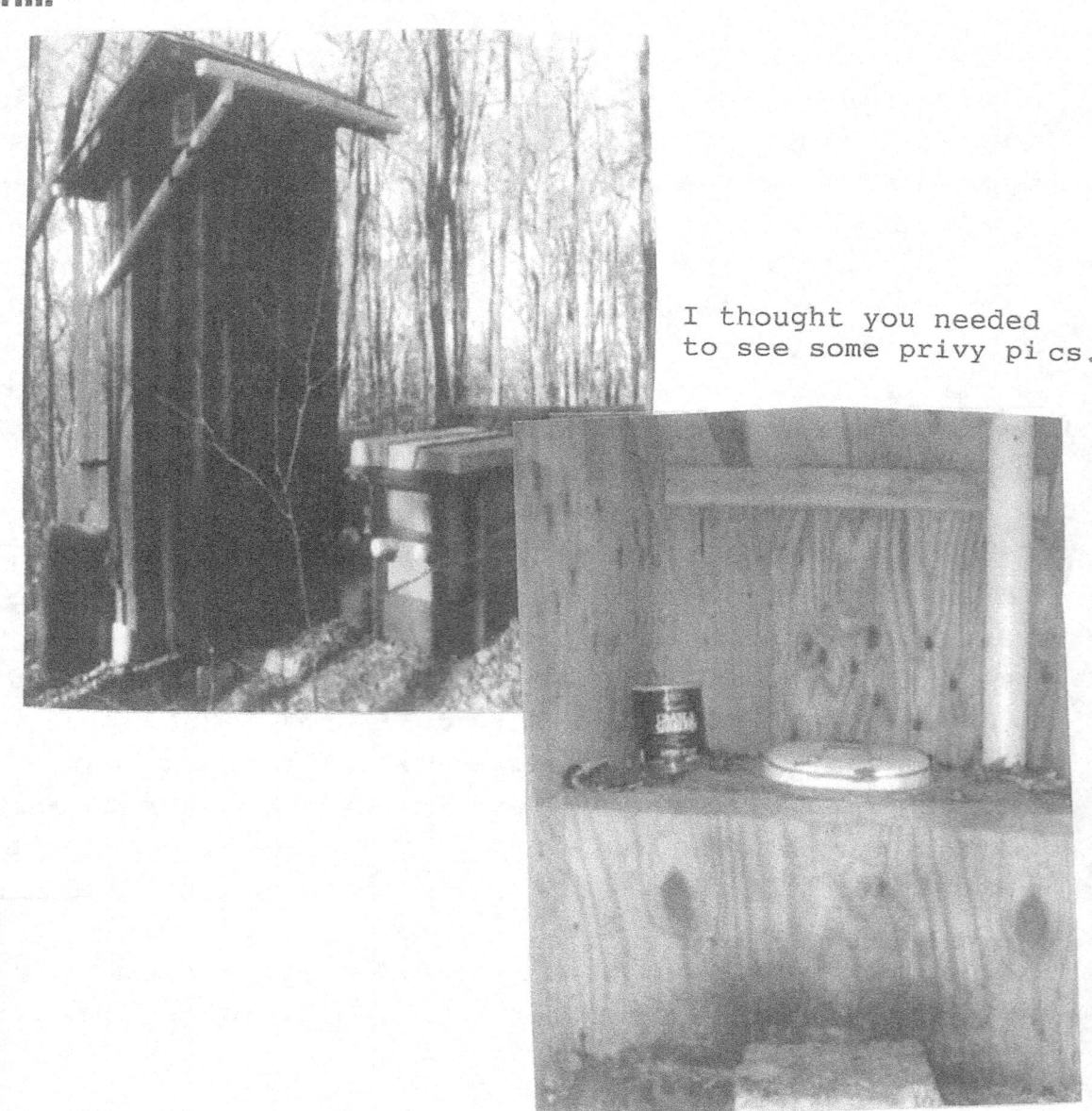

I thought you needed to see some privy pics.

CHAPTER 6
too cold! go home!

One memorable morning I shivered my way out of the tent to go pee. I'd held off all night. I found a proper tree and proceeded to drop my rain pants (for warmth), my hiking pants, my thermal underwear, and of course my underwear and I did what I needed to do. Then, I pulled back on my underwear, my thermal underwear, my hiking pants, and rain pants, and I did this all quickly mind you, and I looked down at the ground that I had just pee'd on and I saw that it had frozen!

Well, you guessed it ...we have opted off the trail for now and will resume in April. It wasn't really that hard of a decision for me anyway. Rex wanted to continue until our snow shoes wouldn't take anymore. (no we didn't actually have snow shoes) Actually it was miserably cold and windy only to keep getting worse. We were going over the Shenandoahs and all of the Skyline Drive restaurants/camping etc had closed for the winter and basically there weren't any other hikers around to speak of.

We would have 5 days or so with out stopping in at any towns. We really wanted to use the lean-tos because it was so windy and cold we felt we needed some form of shelter along with our tent and that would make for some low mileage days due to the spacing apart of the shelters. Sometimes we'd do a fifteen mile a day because a twenty mile day was a bit too much. If we'd try to push to the next shelter inevitably the last few miles would be pure hell. Maybe we could have done big miles but I couldn't bank on it and there wouldn't be any help if we needed it. It was so cold that a lot of the night I laid shivering in the tent and the next day brought relief so long as I kept moving. Which was a great motivator. So, basically I said "take me home for the holidays!".

And so when the decision had finally been made we decided to go home slowly and adjust a little and add some more to our adventure by taking a train ride home. Rex has always been fond of trains and has been on quite a few train rides.

First we used a car rental to get us to Harpers Ferry, then we took the MARC train into Washington D.C. and picked up the Amtrak to Florida about 6 hours later. We had just enough time to poke around DC a little before catching the train. This was my first time being on a train for any real amount of time and I'd never been in a "sleeper" before. When we got into the sleeper I had to snicker at the way that every inch of space was utilized. I'd been in a cruise cabin and felt that they had fully utilized the space but this sleeper had it beat! Once we got settled in I realized that it was roughly the size of the tent but with an upstairs.

After dinner we set up the beds and cuddled up looking out the window. This was really great but being very tired and seriously cramped I said "I love you" as I climbed up to the upper bunk. I felt like a kid in my own clubhouse up there. The nervousness that I'd felt earlier due to the movement of the train went away and I decided to rock with the train as an unborn child does its mother. LOUD doesn't begin to explain all the noise of the train and blowing its horn. I didn't care and slept thru it all.

MAIL..oh yeah! We'd had our mail brought into the house for us and it sat on the kitchen table in a pile waiting for us. I wasn't concerned as I'd been monitoring our accounts and banking online. Well, the things that you couldn't think of happening! We had checks waiting for us from some bank that I was unfamiliar with and I asked Rex "do we have an account with these people" and he said "no, not unless they bought out so and so". Well we each had an account with a local branch that offered $50. for opening up an account. Well, that little account that we each had got purchased by another bank and we had letters from the new bank stating that they were now charging for an account with a balance below their minimum and we now were in default and owed them money. What the heck!

Next, the credit union that we had been using got us. I transferred our account to a more widely used bank that offered clear online banking that I was used to using. A month and a half prior to our leaving I made the change and observed that the online banking with the credit union had seized as I commanded and I picked it up with the newer bank. Well, the credit union did stop the auto payment from coming out of the account for the first month but tried to send it out twice a month for the next 2 months. Each time incurring charges to us as there weren't enough funds to cover. To make it better, the payee decided to charge us for each time the C.U. initiated a payment and then stopped it. Can it get any better? Of course it can! The Credit Union coincidently started using a newer system but "no mistakes were made during the change". Yea right!

Rex received notice that his drivers license was to be revoked. WHAT! We had put our car insurance on a special "we ain't even driving it" plan where we could keep the vehicles legally tagged but we would not be driving them. When Rex's insurance plan came up for renewal it reverted back to the prior coverage and now the lower payments that we were making automatically didn't cover us and we were in default. Fortunately we had found out and corrected this. I went online and found out that the DMV had cleared him. I was about to snap! I needed to run away go back on the trail ASAP. Well, we've got all of it squared a way but it made for a very stressful time. Now, I was stressing and allergy attacking just like the good ole days! (more sarcasm)

I am glad that we have stopped, not just because of the weather but we have more trail to look forward to doing. It is not the end. Not yet. We will return in the spring and savor every moment knowing that it doesn't last forever. Or does it? While we most likely won't be out for such a long time we have many many short trips we have been pondering. We'll see if I feel "talkative" again.

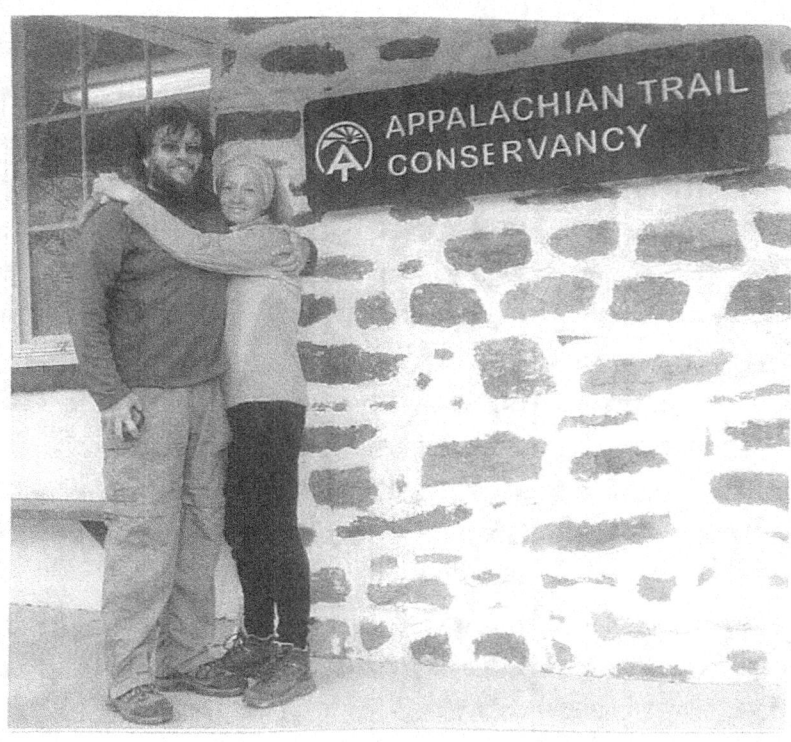

The ATC in Harpers Ferry

CHAPTER 7
BACK ON THE TRAIL

We are in Elkton, VA. now. Our adventure has restarted. The train ride back up to DC went fine excepting it was a few hours late due to severe weather causing trees to fall and block the track. Because we got in late we had to stay in Harpers Ferry after taking the MARC train from DC into town. It was nice to stop by the Appalachian Trail Conservancy again and to stop back in at the Inn. We checked to see if a man whom we'd met at the conservancy was working again. His name is Pop-tart, or Dave T.. He wasn't working today but we saw Barbara who works at the Inn and we bumped into a man that we had met back at the Mohican. We then rented a car and headed to Front Royal. After getting ourselves re-supplied we headed back to the trail.

I had been warned by another hiker that the first part of the trail we were to go across would be a challenge as it goes straight up for hours. But I was determined not to be intimidated any further. Well we got hiking and wow! It was great and not nearly as difficult as I had anticipated. No problem. I was invincible! Then we set up our tent in the lean to for added protection. The next day we set off and I could have just kept on hiking til Georgia. This would be easy. Well, the temperature got up to 82 degrees! What! We were sweating to death and tearing off layers of clothes. Now I really wished that we had stopped at the last stream. We were out of water and felt like we would keel over. Even Rex was dying. And he runs around in a wool uniform out in the heat during Civil War re-enactments. He has been a Florida person his whole life. He was raised with no A/C. He too was ready to drop.

I suggested that he take off one of his outer layers and I stuffed in between his "packa" (raincoat/pack cover) and his pack. Well, it fell out and we lost the fleece that we had purchased in Pinkham Notch. It was an LL BEAN, AMC fleece with so many memories attached. I dropped my pack and went light footed back over a mile of trail and back down but couldn't find it. We got up to the next road and I tried the cell phone. It worked and we were getting picked up. I'd had enough for one day.

Pam at Luray, VA was a God send and knew everyone in town. I mailed home some of our winter things to make our packs lighter. I found out the next day that the temperature was 30 degrees hotter than normal!

Back on the trail we were freezing at night until we got all settled in.   We stayed two nights at Luray while my legs were healing. The boots have torn up both my heals this time and my right knee is trying something new; the painful type of thing. The morning we went back on trail I was sick to my stomach at the restaurant where we ate breakfast. (For several days in a row I have been feeling worse than normal in the morning. I thought "no way!" I can't be having morning sickness. Rex and I are past that time in our lives. I would have to name the child Anthony Thomas. That way we could call the kid A.T.. Hopefully it would be a boy. (ha ha)

Rex left me right along the Skyline drive while he re-traced a few miles of trail; again looking for the lost garment to no avail. If any of you out there, yes you, reading this book, are the person who found this lost garmet, I'll gladly purchase it from you. It was two tones of blue and a size large. Anyway, we kept going and tented in the lean-to that night. Hiking again the next day and it was to rain the following day. Well we stopped in at the Skyline restaurant and the hostess offered us a ride into town. SURE! Sounds great!

On the ride into town, as we drove around and around and down and down into town the hostess told us about some of her hiking experiences and told us about some of the photos that she had taken. She sounded like a real pro.

We'll stop back in on Pam who also worked at the motel in addition to running taxi service. This time in town I bought a knee stable-izer that goes over and around the whole knee. It does seem to help a lot. The most miles we've done so far this time on the trail is 16. It is taking some time to get my legs back. The trail is so easy compared to what we've been through. My head says I should run over it. My legs are saying " oh no you don't". Today we are dodging more bad weather and I am healing my blistered feet and my knees. At this rate, we'll finish around October!

Once again, I need to calm down and not get frustrated. The time spent healing is well spent. It is too easy to underestimate the power of a good nights sleep or time spent allowing your body to recuperate. When we get back on the trail I will want to go like a crazy person again no doubt. Thank God Rex is as patient as can be. When my knee is acting up I go slow like an old lady. Going down is what really hurts. Going up is o.k. Lateral is always great but rare.   The mountains have had snow/ ice on them in spots. All the trees have buds and there are little flowers along the way here and there that are encouraging me " come on! Lets go!" I can't really wait to get back on the trail and see what the mountains are doing. It is beautiful.

Virginia is said to be a green tunnel for hikers as they can't see outside of the trees. With only buds on the trees, we can see clearly. Except for the day that it stayed cloudy all day long. We were hiking along and saw a small group of hikers on a rock overhang. It looked like a rock with trees on either side and a white sheet draped behind the rock. I imagine it was probably quite a drop from there. "Great view" I joked as we hiked by.

One more reason why we get off trail when it's lousy out. Whats the point?

pictures to follow next time we stop

We got a ride in to Elkton from Bob who owns a local motel. There was not a whole lot nearby to say the least. There was a gas station and convenience store that really didn't have a whole lot of what we were hoping for as far as re supply.

We hadn't originally planned to stay in Elkton but our supply is low. We will hang out in Elkton for another two nights and then try to get into Waynesboro quickly. In an attempt to be light packed we hadn't packed enough. It is such a difficult balance trying to pack enough so that you are not "tanking out", as Rex puts it, and carrying too much and being dragged down by the additional weight.

Back when we were thinking about coming thru the Skyline area in the winter (and all the Skyline restaurants and campgrounds would be closed) Bob was a nice guy who answered his phone promptly and said that he'd pick us up at the trail. Would he be willing to pick us up now when business was presumably better?

Yep! Bob came and got us and offered us a ride into town the next day. At the convenience store right nearby we bought up the last of the fried chicken that they had and a breakfast sandwich and some vitamin water and sodas. No denatured alcohol or in-line fuel mix to be had. We took Bob up on his offer into town and he dropped us off at a good place for breakfast. We had things to do. Laundry wasn't one of them as I had hand washed our few clothes and hung them by the heater to dry. We needed fuel, to go to library to update y'all, and we were on the hunt for a new "leatherman" pocket knife; a mini one that has scissors etc. Where ours was I had no idea but knew it would show up eventually.

We wanted some real food to take with us. Some of that chicken that comes in a pouch just like the tuna and some tortilla/burritto wraps and packets of mayonnaise. Well we did have a very good breakfast and we made it to the library, (couldn't download groups of pictures) got some fuel, and were making our way to the grocery store when we stopped in at one of our bank branches to check up on a few things.

The nice bank manager told us about a man just across the street who was a local historian. So of course off we went and visited he and his wife at their business, a TV repair shop, and they looked busy. Who knows what all else they fixed but they had parts and TV s dating back. It was his Dad's business who sold it to them. They told us where to walk to go see a hospital, Jennings Hospital, that Stonewall Jackson marched his troops past and also a home that Stonewall used as his headquarters. Stonewall's wife joined him there and this is called the Miller-Argabright-Cover-Kite House. Now when I go back and read thru some of Rex's gazillian books about the Civil War some of this will ring a little bell in my head as I'll be able to recall having been there. There are so many historical places that we've been to and thru. This was a nice surprise.

We stopped in on the local bbq joint in hope of some good "Q" for Rex. To no avail this was another crock pot kind of bbq joint. Nice people though.

It was beautiful to walk across the Shenandoah River (with out a pack on). The towns of Elkton and Luray all had beautiful spring flowers popping up everywhere. Up on the trail I would see these white flowers with 5 petals and then I'd see an occasional bright red one. Silly bright red; such bright red that when hiking I thought I was looking at a reflector, the kind you could have along the side of the driveway. When I got upon it I realized it was a flower! Then there were all these bright green leaves growing out of the ground in little clumps. A few times I saw white or pink flowers popping out and I 'd look around and think "wow!". When these all pop out it will be crazy. And we did come thru a few areas where they had all bloomed and it was crazy beautiful. I saw these short little flowers, Irises? And then I saw a few Pink Lady Slippers. I remembered them from my walks thru the woods with my Mom when I was just a girl and she'd tell me 'Don't pick one. They are endangered".

The views that we have had off the side of the mountains are unbelievable. Virginia is a place where thru hikers have a hard time. Traditionally the hiker comes thru Virginia when everything is all green and you can't see anything but what is directly in front of you. For us everything is budding and just beginning to bloom so we can clearly see over the sides of the mountains. It's hard to go too far with out a picture perfect view. It is times like this that I am grateful for this extra time on the trail. If we had pushed through we would have missed out on so much!

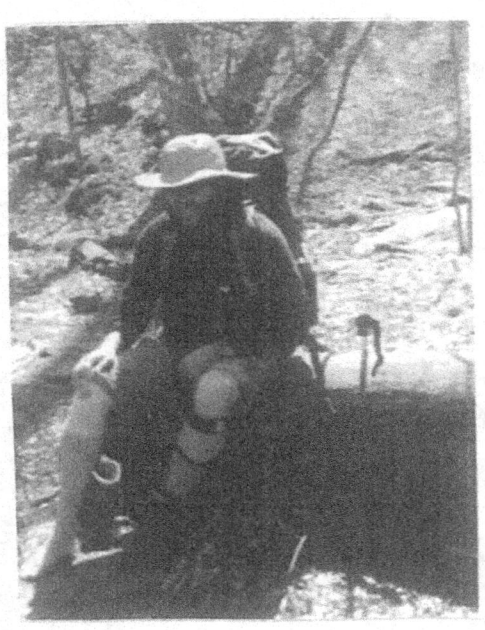 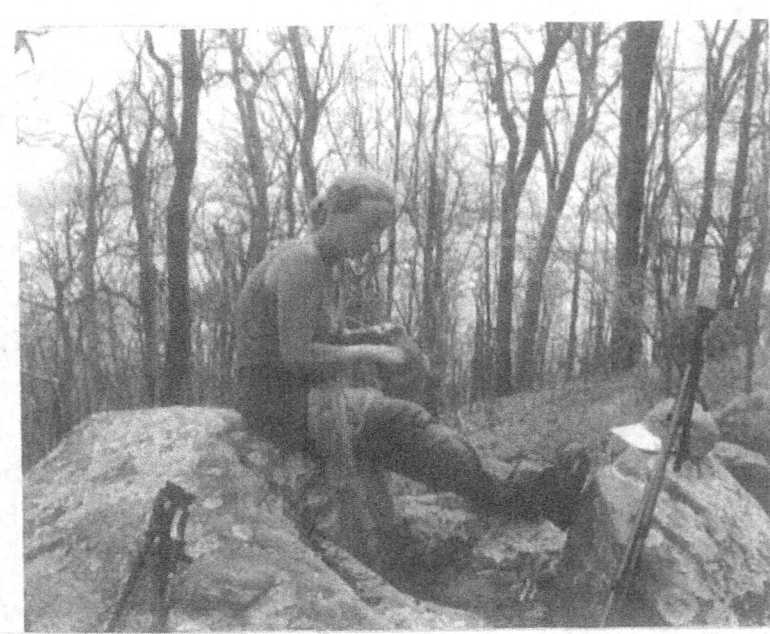

Rex's knee shows signs of things to come.

Waynesboro, VA! We couldn't wait. We'd been told we needed to go to a particular restaurant. Are we on the Appalachian Trail or a restaurant tour? We ducked into Waynesboro for my birthday April 16th which was also predicted to be raining.

Good timing.   Well, rain it did all day long. We went to the outfitter there, a great place, and we spent hours. We bought Rex another pair of pants, we found a mini leatherman!, and a compression bag. His boots totally blew out and were flapping in the breeze and I said "just wait I'm calling that manufacturer" then Rex reminded me of how long he'd had the boots and how many miles he'd put on them. Gee it didn't seem that long ago to me. Then for me; a new pair of socks for my birthday! (Rex had already gotten me an early gift before we came out) We went for bbq in town it was good bbq! The sweet tea you could stand your spoon up in it even after it was diluted some for us.   We went to the local Italian restaurant for my birthday. This was an old fashioned sit down kind of place. Great food! I got chic parm (original hu?) and Rex got something with mushrooms and all. We were both real pleased and for the time being we were not feeling hungry.

The next day I'd arranged a ride from a trail angel we'd heard of thru the outfitters. The "older couple" (what really is "old"?) came and picked us up right on time and took us to where we'd gotten off trail. The man had done the trail a few years back. The trail angels lived on the mountain and said that they had never seen so much rain and that we had a total of 8 inches of rain. They had managed to squeeze us in before church that Sunday.

Again we were back on the trail and every stream that we came to was over burdened with water gushing down. What would normally be a simple crossing was now much more difficult. We'd have to examine the best way of getting across. Many times we opted to just take off our boots and wade thru. It was better than risking a wet boot all day or getting pulled down the river as I did in Maine. We'd go across fallen logs when we could. It was nerve racking to me. Somedays we only did 13 miles; like when we went up the Priest Mountain. Other times we did 20 or more.

On Easter Sunday we hiked about 18 and got to a lousy shelter ... lousy because it had no water, never did.There was a man there that Rex didn't feel real comfy being around so we hiked another 3 miles or so to get into Buchanon. These extra three miles really seemed to take their toll on us but Rex wanted us to sleep in a bed for Easter. I was tired and didn't really care if I slept propped against a tree but onward we went and got out to where we could hitch into town. That is if anybody was out there to give us one.

So, we stood waiting for someone to drive by and swatting at gnats and two young guys came by to offer us a lift. These guys were definitely "on something". It always makes me a little bit nervous when here you've been hiking day in and day out and you get into a car and whoooosh you are off. Driving along the side of a mountain with the road weaving in and out. EVERYONE is doing 50 MPH and you wonder what if the brakes went bad? Well they've got that figured! There are run-away-truck places built into the sides of the mountain where you can just go weeeeeeeeeeehh.... right up the side of the mountain till you stop. Oh my gosh!

So these two guys give us a ride into town and we turn left and run out of town. I call the motel and some lady tells me which way to go. We drive thru town and onto the interstate and off again at the first exit. Oh great! "This won't be hard to get back onto trail" I think sarcastically. We offered the guys some gas money for going the extra distance for us and we were off to get a room and go to the restaurant on the same property. Well the room we got. The restaurant was not yet open for the season. What!!!

We hiked down the really big hill to the gas station/convenience store. Our knees ached and our legs were screaming at us. "What would you like for dinner" I asked looking at the hot dogs that had been going for a ride on the carousel for how long?   I knew this wouldn't be good. But at least we had the Celebrity Apprentice to look forward to watching. We got 3 of those prepackaged hamburgers and some other junk and back to our room we went. I wasn't going to think about how we'd get back on the trail and if it took all day I'd just have to deal with it. We micro-waved the burgers in the motel office and the Apprentice was about to begin! The burgers were surprisingly good! We pulled down the bedspread and blanket and sat on top of the sheet but not under the sheets we'd take a shower after we'd eaten and watched the show. We both stank. Well I know I sure did. Which may be part of the reason why we had not seen many bears. They'd get a whiff of me and stay away.

After we showered we had a little hiker sex. That's where you get on the bed with your head to the others feet and give each other a foot rub. What were you expecting?!! ha ha

The next morning we were back off to the gas station and down the long hill. I asked the man there if there were any taxi's in the area. I knew the answer already, but what the heck? Is this what they call fishing? Then I told him that we'd been real lucky and got a ride into town last night but now it would be difficult to make our way back onto the trail. "Is it even be legal to try and hitch off the interstate?" I asked him.

I may have grumped about the restaurant being closed too. So, this guy that I had assumed was just a minimum wage earner told us that he owned the motel and the gas station and the restaurant and if we went back up the hill and got our packs he'd get us a ride into town as he knew everyone that came in there and where they were going. WOW! I guess I casually pissed and moaned in front of the right guy! And with in 12 minutes we had a ride into town! I turned to say thanks and saw him giving us the thumbs up sign. Wow he really saved us. Then in town we stopped in on the Burger King and then easily hitched back to the trail.

The couple that gave us a ride in to town stated that they often had done the same for other hikers. They too were hikers. This is often the case. Some people that picked us up hiking had family members, sons sometimes, that were hikers. Some ride givers seemed lonely. Some wanted to hear all about Rex and I and what we were doing while others just needed to tell us their stories. All of the ride givers were great. We were so appreciative.

On a few different occasions, we'd come thru a tourist type area and people would ask us questions and sometimes even take our picture. Gee! That makes me feel like a move star.

Then we'd meet up with other hikers who claimed to have done the AT before and then they'd say that they had done the Pacific Crest Trail or some other large trail and make us feel like we hadn't done anything.

We stopped also at Glasgow. We just had to as it was too close by not to. Where the trail met the road it was so busy with big trucks and cars whipping down the road and passing each other. Maybe I've lived in Florida too long or maybe I'm getting too old but these people had a death wish. Where could we stand that someone could actually stop? We got a ride into town to find that the restaurant was out of business. We had two convenience stores and a Dollar General. We were in great shape. There was even a canvas sort of shelter thing that some Eagle Scout had made across the street.   One of the stores made sandwiches and had fried chicken. We took 4 or 5 pieces of chicken for a snack while we waited on the large steak and cheese grinder we'd ordered.

With our bellys fat and full we decided to go farther on the trail. We hiked along for a short time and came hiking right past the lean to! This was absolutely incredible! Usually you are nearly in tears to find the next lean to. They never just sneak up on you. I've even gone so far as to start sniffing for a privy in hopes of a lean to near by.

The shelter is right next to a stream. This is perfect. I'm loving the trail at this moment. We set up tent and it rained that night. The tent was wet when we rolled it up. Not that I'm one to complain, but, the tent is my responsibility to carry and it felt like I had a wet towel rolled up with it. We had full bottles of water too. I was dying hiking. How can this be? We've eaten well and we've slept well. The trail was so easy compared to what we've gone thru before. This is crazy. I'm getting discouraged.

That night we camped at another shelter and let the tent completely dry before setting it up. It seems that Rex and I take turns feeling badly. I feel bad every single morning, even sick to my stomach, and Rex is bopping around feeling happy. Then in the afternoon when he gets tired I feel new strength. Well, now it was time for his knees to start hurting. First one knee then the other. I knew about this as I'd been thru it myself. Well one knee was really making things difficult for him. We got him a knee brace and took the next two days at just 10 miles per day. That would put us stopping at the Home Place Restaurant that we'd heard so much about. Everyone told us to make sure that we'd stop there. We did and we were not disappointed.

They offered family style "all you can eat", and that, we did. The owner had told me over the phone that we could tent camp on the property. Did he really mean it? The property was green and beautiful and up on a hill with cows etc fenced out on the sides. Yes, he did mean it and we tent camped right on the side of the restaurant next to a pavilion. At night the property was lit up like a foot ball stadium. Going pee was a bit of a predicament. More on that another time. In the morning I said "o.k. hon, we've got 72 miles till we get to another stop. Should we resupply for 5 or 6 days or for 2 or 3 days or what. Can you go any further?". Rex was in a lot of pain. Sleeping on a hard surface didn't make it any easier, though the grass at the restaurant was the best we'd had so far. He needed a couple days off his feet. Even the 10 mile days weren't helping him any. The "Devil's Tooth" was coming up next. Would it be that bad? We didn't know.

Which brings me to ask...."the Devil's Tooth", "the Priest", "the Guillotine", "Blood Mountain". There were no "Hello Kitten Mountains" or "sure you can do it" mountains. No, every one had a nasty and intimidating name.

So, we landed in Salem, VA and spent a total of 5 nights. We got dropped off at a hotel about 3/4 of a mile away from stores and things. We got a room and went out with out the weight of our packs and walked into town. This put a lot stress on his knee. The next day we changed hotels.

We bought a pair of crutches from the Goodwill next door to keep the weight off of his knee. He was in too much pain. I couldn't slap a pack on his back and tell him to go hike a few mountains and giving him a piggy back ride was not an option. I tried to casually mention the idea of "slack packing". That's when someone drops you off and picks you up at night so that you are not carrying your pack. Again, he said that this was not his style and he probably couldn't physically do that anyway. He was having enough trouble just going across the street. So, after researching our cheapest means of getting home. We rented a car and made it back to his brother's in Jacksonville, FL..

It is hard on us both but especially for Rex. But, our way of doing the trail has never been about "who can endure the most pain". <u>We choose to enjoy the trail</u>. If it rains then we take a day off. If my blisters get too bad then we take a day off. And now, we will stay off trail until Rex is healed. Whats the point in continuing? Just to be miserable the whole time or to possibly do serious damage if it's not done already? So, now we wonder whether or not to see a doctor. Probably we will. I just hope that we get a good one. Know a really great sports medicine doc? A physical therapist that I got to talking to said that she'd go to a neurologist first. Is that the route we should go? Any input will be appreciated. This is a new area for us both. By the time we are done we'll know, no doubt. It is our plan to hopefully be fully healed and able to return to the trail in August. I'd like to leave behind my sleeping bag and just carry a small sheet to start with. We are considering getting those blow up sleeping pads. They sell for about $150. a piece. We've never had the best of luck with blow up beds etc but we've heard people rant about these things. Feel free to offer your input. much more later,

God Bless!

oh yea, I found our original leatherman. It was in my pocket book that I'd left at Rex's brother Butch's.

SIDE NOTE:
Rex was given a round of prednisone by our doctor. That and some rest and he was good to go.

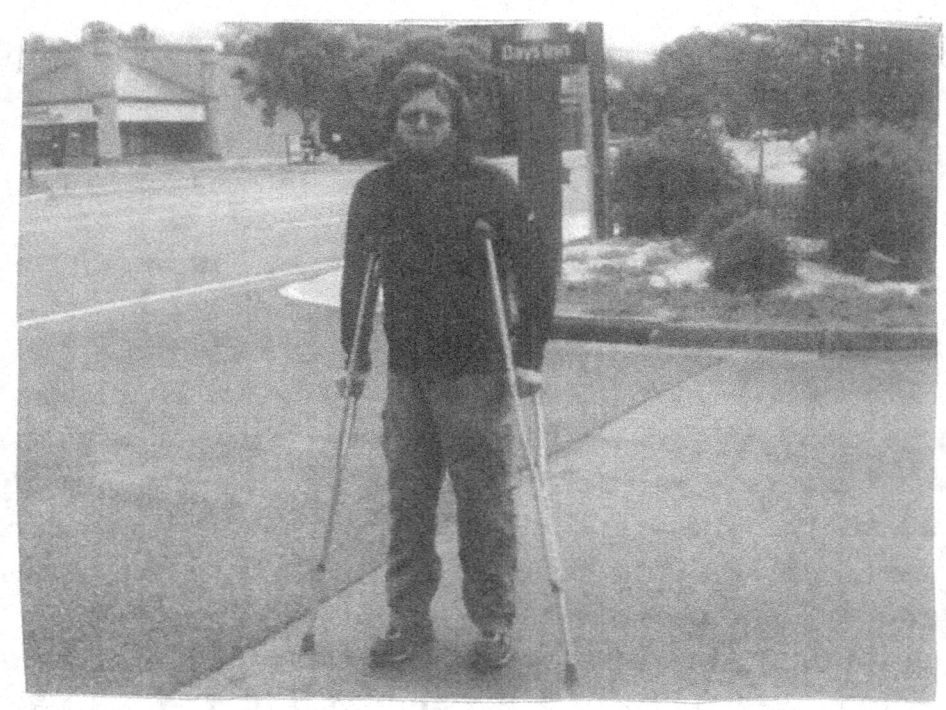

oh no!

CHAPTER 8

Back on the trail once again,

We got on the bus in Macon to return yet again and the bus terminal was interesting as we watched a passenger with his pants totally torn across the back end exposing his rear end and we wondered how that happened. There was a man there that appeared homeless because of his long over grown white beard and unkempt appearance. Off we go to the first of 4 stops. The next stop was really crowded, it was hot and smelled like armpits. Everyone was calm and polite but worn from the heat. There we stood, literally stood, as though waiting for The Great Pumpkin to arrive, for 3 hours. Then a passenger with a smart phone told us we had another hour to go.

I finally sat on the floor with my pack. O.K. you should expect delays. The next stop we were getting off and taking our baggage and the door would not open. After a while the baggage man said "oh, your staying on this bus anyway." O.K. I guess it must be because of the bus being late. We got a new bus driver and made it to our next stop and she told us "now you know that your bus won't be here until 11:30 am." What!

So we sat on these benches that were engineered to be uncomfortable. The benches had partitioning arm sections as not to allow laying down and the seat was made as an oven rack so that the fatty/cushion part of your rear end and legs would get caught in between the grates. I was freezing cold, it was like a meat locker in there. Finally, I decided to put some newspaper under me and that worked well, and I thought "well, I could put some on top of me too!" And I realized, "oh no! that's how it starts. I'll look just like a homeless person"! Well the bus did arrive it was only an hour and a half past "due" time. We eagerly gave them our packs to store in the underneath compartment and we were told to go get something to eat. "But we're not hungry!"; Oh no, the buss had a flat tire.

SALEM, VA yet again

We stayed in Salem for two nights and got caught up on our sleep. Off we went in the morning. We made it about 12 miles although not with out tears. The boots I was wearing, <u>which I had broken in</u>, hurt so bad. But I knew that blisters were bound to happen for me. It's just part of it. I'll get toughened skin and I will deal with it. The next day 10 miles; It was all I could do to crawl those miles. The next day we started hiking and I nearly used the "Q" word. You know it rhymes with "hit". I said I need a day to heal. We stayed at the lean-to for the day. Off we were to go in the morning. We made it to Newport, VA. By now we had used up all of the food that we had to make it to Pearisburg.

The water situation is awe-full right now. Streams are bone dry. We are having to carry extra water (weight). We saved some weight by not carrying our sleeping bags. I felt pretty smart about that. It being August and all we usually just lay in the tent dripping sweat. I was actually happy if Rex let out a fart, just to feel the breeze.

Well in Newport we sat on the side of the road for a while with the few cars that went by just driving on past us, one driver waved to us using just one finger. And then Sandy came by and he offered us a ride. He was going to the store and said he'd even wait for us. WOW great! We hit the jack pot. As not to be a burden for him we ran around the store gathering what we anticipated we'd need and were back in the truck in a jiffy. He offered us to camp outside his house, many a hiker had done it in the past. Cool, O.K.. While we sat making small talk with he and his long time friend Connie, my ankles oozed and stung so bad. I took more Ibuprofin and put more antibacterial salve on them. Our hosts were being so kind to us and I could hardly keep up a conversation. I felt like a bum. I was so grateful to them for all of their kindness. I was in a great deal of pain. My blisters were red and disgusting. Pictures to follow, when I can.

That night we froze our butts off as the temperatures got down to the high 50s. Now I'm not so glad that I didn't bring the sleeping bags.

Rex said "We need to get you new boots.". I said "I can make it if we just go a few miles at a time". But, I was in too much pain to argue. The next day we got a hold of a shuttle provider and off again to Salem, VA. Well, next door in Roanoke as many of you know is a really cool train system. Rex and I killed most of a day at the transportation museum. I love watching Rex's eyes light up like a boys at the trains. We went to another museum and had a great time. Eventually after going everywhere I found a pair of boots.

Connie came and got us at the bus stop when we were returning to the trail. We couldn't stay the night but Connie and her son sent us off with roses. That made us feel pretty special. She is such a nice woman. I hope to see her again.

Back on the trail after 4 nights of healing. Water is scarce. We are getting to places in our book listed as water sources and they are "dry as a popcorn fart" as Rex would say. My heels are killing me still. We are trying everything. Being allergic to adhesives doesn't help me any. Well I stuffed so much foam rubber behind my heals that it hurt my toes. One of my big toes is all blistered under and beneath the nail. I think I'll loose the nail. The trails themselves have been great.

One day I was in so much pain I just sat down on the ground, no comfy rocks around, and cried. I took off my boots and put on the shoes used for around camp and in towns. These are light weight, if you were to mail them- 2 stamps-not more than 3. They are good for going out and getting the mail. The bottoms are soft like a baby's butt, smooth. I put them on and my feet felt great. If feet could smile; mine were smiling. I easily hiked the next 3 miles to the lean-to. Only to find out that there was no water. We hiked to the next marked campsite with water; no water. We went to bed without our usual Ramen noodles. We each had a liter of water to get us through the night and the next day to another place 3 miles further that supposedly had water.

The next morning; no water. We hiked a little further and found a spring in between the rocks; YES WATER!

Well, the good part is WE SAW BEAR. Yes I can finally say "we saw bear". It seems to be the only thing that anybody cares about as everyone always asks us "have you seen any bear?". I always felt a little ripped off that we hadn't seen any bear but I'd rather have it that way than seeing a grumpy bear up close.

Now we resupply again and plan to only go 8 to 10 miles per day until my heel situation gets better. We will have much better opportunity for re-supplying the next 60 or so miles.

So, ALL of you who said you'd like to join us....NOW is the time! Come have fun with us. And please, bring a cold ginger ale for Rex and a cold orange soda for me, with some ice please.

DAMASCUS

THIS IS BIG!!! We have made it to DAMASCUS, VA! Not only are we only 3 miles from being out of Virginia but Damascus is a big place for hikers as they host the annual Trail Days every June. We wanted to be here for the hiker days but obviously too many other things happened. So things are going better! My feet are making friends with my boots; that is, after loosing a few toe nails etc. Sometimes I'll hike 8 - 10 miles and then switch over to my bedroom slipper type sandals and hike another 6 to 8 miles.

We have recently come through the Grayson Highlands State Park where there are wild ponies. We went through a gate and were greeted by fat little ponies looking for carrots. Gee I thought, " this is more like a petting zoo". Later after hiking up and over every rocky high land they have we left through the gate and a mile or so later I was surprised to see ponies just hanging out by themselves.

We have been having such an adventure. It has been painful and rewarding to look back on. We have met other hikers that have been real nice. One hiker asked if I'd used the privy at the previous lean to. I said no but I'd seen the sign that said 'Nice Privy". It looked to me like it had been torn down and only had the steps remaining and a plastic bucket or something on top. He explained that on top was a toilet. It was out in the open. This he found to be refreshing, and not stinky as the usual privy, and he dropped his drawers and took a poop right there. He was rewarded with a deer coming by to see him.

Sleep has been extra hard for me. There has been an eery feeling; hardly any hikers and no water. We've been told that wild animals are coming into residential areas for water. There are no bubbling springs or running streams to sleep by. Every night I hear bears and deers come by the tent. They will grunt at each other and push things around. I often hear coyotes. One night there was a hiker's head light around our tent at 2am. I was scarred to death. There was only a single male hiker, nice guy, in the lean to when we went to bed. Who was this that was around the outside of our tent? I nearly pee'd myself. After a little bit of time I literally had to pee. The light was further away and I got up and saw 2 headlamps setting up their tent on the other side. What creeps I thought. The next morning while walking past their tent I commented about not getting any sleep and I clanged my hiking sticks together loudly. For three nights in a row I had really bad nightmares.

So we got to a visitors center the next day and spoke with a nice forest ranger/sheriff about the water situation. He looked up on his fancy maps to try and help us to determine the best chances of water. Then he asked us some questions. Here we learned about a murder on the trail. A male and female couple were suspects. oh no! Were we "supects"? No, We didn't fit in the same age group as the suspects. But based on what we were told, it may have been them, the suspects, that came around our tent at 2am. Oh Great! We'll never get another ride into town once word gets out about this!

SLEEP DEPRIVATION AND POTTY TALK

Since we have been back again on the trail the water situation has been really bad. Where there is normally a raging stream the size of a lane of traffic it is now all dried up. We have been carrying extra water and hoping that the water sources listed in our book are there. We know that some springs above 2500 feet will be dry and streams too. There is a large river that runs through this area but it is cow pastures and we have come to the conclusion and also been told by others that it would not be wise to use this water even though we ALWAYS use sterilization procedures. One time we used questionable water but we boiled it before we used it.

So we will go about 10 miles a day due to my feet and we always try to stop for the night at a water source.

One time we came into Big Walker Gap and there was a piped spring that took an hour and 20 minutes to fill a 1 liter bottle of water. So we just camped right there for the night as the water was good and just kept filling our bottles and left the next morning with full bottles to see how far we could get.

I planned our next miles to involve a stop at a restaurant when we came by a town and the next day we would stop at a shelter next to a visitors center. Well it was only 8 miles to get to the restaurant but then we'd have time to hitch into town and resupply and hitch back out etc. Well the book wasn't very clear to me but we came out on the trail right at the restaurant! Finally a break. WOW great!

We'd gotten up early and I was leading us as fast as I could. We got there at 10:30 am just in time for breakfast. I asked if we could tent site any where close by and I was told sure you can camp right here and I was shown an area around the side and back of the restaurant that was built up to be the same height as the front (we were on a mountain, you know) There is a skirted area built up off the parking area where we are told to tent so that no trucks or cars could run us over. So I'm thinking, we caught a break today and got into town without hitching etc. Its about time things start going my way. I'm just sitting my happy little ass here where there is food and water and tomorrow we will hike into the Partnership Shelter by the visitor center where we can order pizza for dinner. This is more of my idea of rouging it.

We set up our tent after having dinner and at 8pm the restaurant closed. If you married people have ever played the farting under the sheets and stinking out your spouse game then you could appreciate how bad it was being in a hot little tent that night. Tonight Rex was winning this stink contest. Again, we were lit up like a football stadium, but I didn't care. I snuck a pee behind the restaurant under a down spout and made a mental note to pour water over it in the morning and we went to "bed".

Soon after I heard an 18 wheeler pull in. Well, I'm glad that we are up here not to be run over. And I drifted off to sleep. Not too long later I awoke hearing in my head a song that I hadn't heard in a long long time..... chhhhurch (radio crackle) this here is rubber duck...we have us a convoy! Yes, we've got a little convoy rocking through the night...come and see our convoy, aint' she a beautiful site...la la la la la convoy..scubby doobey doo... OK so I don't remember exactly all the words but you remember it. I peered outside the tent and saw ten 18 wheelers facing towards us! Their motors of course are all still on and their compressors periodically making sounds.

After a few days on the trail and eating big in town and your stomach is not your friend. I awoke all of a sudden with the earth moving beneath me. This time it wasn't an earthquake. I had to "go"...like now! So I awoke Rex and told him I was going across the highway to the gas station bathroom. He didn't like the idea of me parading past all the truckers and across the highway to a gas station bathroom at 2am by myself and so he escorted me.

There is a woman stocking cigarettes at the store and I ran by and said "good morning", as not to startle her, and when I came out I said "how you doing?". Rex who had been sitting on a bench waiting for me said "lets go". Come to find out, the lady was all upset about my using the bathroom and it was just for customers and called her boss to get permission to put a closed sign on the door and yah deee yah dee yah. She'd asked Rex if we were "walking" and he said that we were staying at the restaurant across the street. Where did she think we hikers bought our resupply from? I'm NOT a homeless person. I am a hiker! Anyway...the life of a hiker.

****

Hey that reminds me of this joke:

Whats the difference between a hiker and a homeless man?
Give up?
Goretex! ha ha

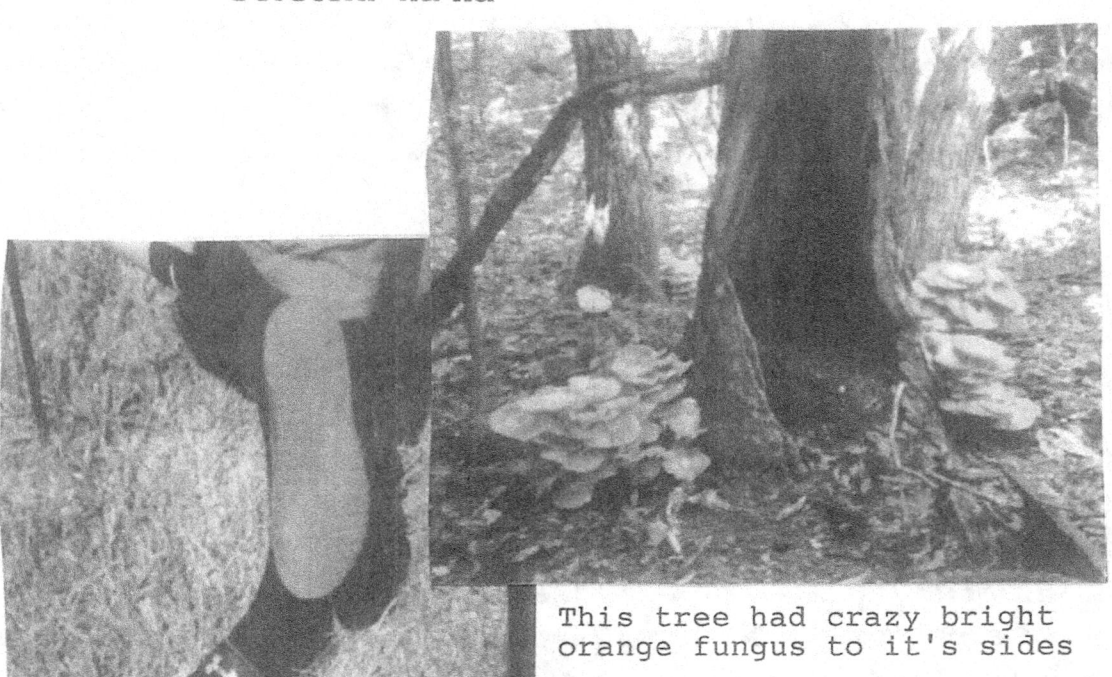

This tree had crazy bright
orange fungus to it's sides

Colleen's shoes

Rex has been tormented by bees and wasps getting stung every couple of days. To make matters worse, last night sitting in front of the hostel under a light, all of a sudden a moth flew in under Rex's hair and directly into his ear. He tilted his head and started talking loudly and banging on his head. I told him to tilt his head the other way, facing up, and I put a hiker headlight on his ear to coax it out. Moths are attracted toward light, right? By now he was trying really really hard to remain calm as the thing was flying around in his head where it could not even be seen. Eventually it came toward the light and when I could I grabbed it by its little wings and I saw that it had a 3 inch wingspan! Poor Rex can't get that feeling "out of his head"! ha ha

One night we got water from a house nearby, it was a nice man who even gave us some peaches from his tree and we hobo camped just off the road. My step mom texted us to see if we were ok with something about an earthquake? I called back and was surprised to learn that the epicenter of the earthquake was really close to where we where. We'd been about 30 miles away from the epicenter. "No we hadn't felt a thing" I told her. I didn't have any bad dreams after that.   Rex thinks that I could feel something coming on. He describes it kinda like the zoo animals! Who knows.

Oh yeah, the *other* national disaster(!), I nearly forgot. After spending the night filling our water bottles we hiked up to an enclosed shelter. It was a fire watchers/caretakers shelter up on top of a mountain with no trees around it. The structure got a new roof in about 1995 and it had steel cables to secure it. This is where we would wait out the storm. I took a camera phone picture of Rex next to the shelter to show my concerned family that we'd be OK. I convinced my Dad that we were in no harm of a flash flood. (we were at 4400 feet) My sister also saw the picture and said she was calling the National Guard. Apparently the shelter didn't reassure her. I told her that we were safe but the room service was slow.
If Rex asks "what else could go wrong" one more time I'm going to have to hurt him. ha ha
SORRY pictures wont work here..we've got lots to share though.

WE HAVE PICS NOW!! We are in HOT SPRINGS, NC ! Only 271.8 more miles to go. I have gone ahead thru our book and tried to figure our daily miles and resupply etc and I am thinking that we should be able to make it into Springer Mountain for Rex's B-day which is Oct. 15th. We are at the library right now and we have an excellent librarian who has been trying to help us use the batch option for downloading pictures to no avail. Not even with her sneaky-do passwords and all. So, Rex is painstakingly single photo downloading for all to enjoy and so that we have photos stored online in case we both fall down into a river or something.

My head is about to explode right now as I've just gotten off the computer where I was checking our bank account and I've learned that a couple of things have gotten messed up despite my doing everything humanly possible to have them taken care of in advance. But I've got it squared away now.

Hiking this trail has cost far more than anticipated! I forget exactly where I've left off. What I'd like to blog goes thru my head as we hike and I don't really remember if I've actually written it or not.

So, last we were in Pearisburg and so much has happened since then.   It has been so difficult getting into Pearisburg for me. The streams were dry. The springs were dry. And of course there was my never ending blisters.

The Chestnut Knob Shelter has windows and a door. Inside there was a picnic table and a couple of platforms for sleeping. Rex and I were making ourselves at home. We unpacked and I changed into my long johns. We decided to put up our tent inside to stay warm and we found a spot to hang our food. We figured we'd have the place to ourselves and in walked a young male hiker. He spoke with an English accent. I didn't know if he could be trusted or not. After talking for a bit I determined that he was o.k.. When he mentioned a hiker that he'd shared a shelter with in the past I couldn't believe it because Rex and I also knew this hiker from a different year. That's the trail for you.

We couldn't get any water at one lean to and we headed into a hostel that was a short distance away. By now whenever my feet would act up I'd take out my little slippers. We easily hiked in the remaining 4.8 miles in and hour and 45 minutes. The young couple who owned the hostel were going on vacation in a few days and it rather showed that they were in need of a vacation. It was not the "wonderful place" we'd thought it would be. They did have water, at least kind of. Their pigs had tripped the automatic water system and the spring had run dry leaving us with no showers that night. I didn't really need one as it had only been 4 or 5 days. ha ha

The hiker area consisted of mattresses tossed on the floor one next to another in the loft. There were no mattress covers etc. I wouldn't let my dog stay there.

When we stayed at a motel in Pearisburg I accidently left the key in the room. So, I went around to the front where there was a sign "working around back". I went around the back and found no one there so I called the owner by phone and he answered the phone and I told him my dilemma and he said "oh..well I'm in *West* Virginia" .What! I guess when everyones in for the night he goes off and does his stuff. So there we were with no car (obviously), sitting outside the motel overhang waiting for the rain to start. We didn't know if we should go get another motel room or what. The owner told me over the phone that room 28 had the same key as ours. The man staying in there had a black truck. Room 28, we would sit and wait for him to return. He should be back soon we were told. "What if he decides to stay out all night long?" I thought. Finally it occurred to me, something from my detective childhood days, and I used a credit card to pop open our door. So much for security.

We stayed at the Troutdale Baptist Church hostel which was really cool. It had showers and a pump with a clothes line for doing our laundry. Not to mention Jerry's Restaurant! We loved this place! The owner could not have been any nicer to us and he gives all of his guests a ride back to the trail.

We stayed in Damascus as the trail goes right thru town. I got a little discouraged at a couple of hikers that we met there. One was a 30 year old going on the trail for his second time and he'd slack packed his way the first time. Now he had quit his job and mom was paying for the trail for him.

There seem to be more than a few of these bums. But then we've met recently a couple of young and really "with-it" hikers that were philosophical and spiritual and made me feel like a bum because lately my attitude hasn't been all that it should and I'm ready to get this done with already.

Stinky Feet and More Hygiene

Lets talk about our feet here for a moment. When we were going thru Massachusetts one of the things that I really was concerned about was having dry socks.

A cold night is even colder with out any dry socks. I'd been told that if you have dampish clothing that it will dry out over night if you wear it inside your sleeping bag with you. This never worked for me.

Sometimes I will use a safety pin and I'll attach my socks to the back of my back pack so that they can dry during the day. I recall coming thru the white mountains with socks blowing behind my pack.

My feet get so stinky that my family decided to Google this for me so that we might learn the cause. One explanation for the ammonia type odor was from being dehydrated. The other explanation was that the person is burning protein, not fat. I don't know if I have ever got so skinny that I was burning protein but who knows. Not drinking enough; I know that I am guilty.

My socks sometimes will become so acidic that wearing them for more than one day is not a good option. Sometimes my feet will get a sort of acid burn. I try to drink enough but it is not always easy.

When we were up in Baxter State Park the ranger, Betty, told us to soak our legs in the streams to remove the acidic acid that builds up. I could do this for a short time but it was too cold for me. I don't know how Rex did it, but he did.

When the weather is cooler I often times don't realize how dehydrated I've gotten. It becomes such an inconvenience to stop and take off your pack to pee. When you are hiking you get hot and don't need a lot of clothing. When you stop you need to immediately cover yourself so that you don't get hypothermia.

Think of the athletes that you see on T.V. with their warm up jackets on when they are not playing.

During the warmer season I could just slide my shorts aside and not even have to take off my pack or pull down my pants. With the cooler weather, I have to stop and drop my back pack and drop my drawers. It gets cold and takes up time

At night I hate to drink anything because I'll have to climb out of the warm tent into the cold.

When Rex and I get into town we just can't get enough to drink. Rex, and we've heard from many others, don't usually drink carbonated beverages (sodas) but will absolutely crave them while hiking. Rex goes crazy for a cold ginger ale!

I was asked what has been the longest period of time between showers for me. I think the longest period of time with out a shower and soap has been about 15 days. In Maine during the summer, we'd rinse ourselves in a stream when we could.

Initially, I carried a full stick of deodorant and I used it in the morning and at night. I quickly learned that I was building up a thick layer of deodorant and it was holding in the sweat and the stink that comes along. I learned to go with out deodorant and to allow myself to dry out as much as I could.

We've learned to never carry a full roll of toilet paper. I'll take about a half of a roll with out the cardboard in the center.

As far as toothpaste, I'll buy a trial size and let some go down the drain so that I am only carrying half. It weighs too much you know!

This trail has totally changed my thinking. Shopping at the warehouse stores, buying in bulk, and shopping for the best prices are all things that we do on a normal basis. The trail has me looking for the smallest available amount.

Some store and hostels will sell small quantities to hikers. Items are purchased and repackaged. Powdered drinks are often repackaged into small plastic bagfulls.

We always carry our toothbrushes but don't use them nearly as frequently as we do at home.

I am always seeking a disposable razor and a few Qtips when we get to a shower.

I carry one hair pick type of comb with me. This is good enough to get thru any snarled hair we may have.

One memorable evening, Rex and I were at our camp spot and I was setting up our tent while Rex was cooking and "roping a bear tree'.   Well when he came into the tent with the evenings piping hot wonderful Ramen noodles, he said "oh no!", "we've set our tent up right where someone's pooped!". "No" I said. "It's your hiking boots under the vestibule of the tent.".

Placing the boots under the vestibule has been convenient to allow them to dry, but they do somewhat smell. Putting them at the foot of the tent isn't much better because your clothes and sleeping bag are in close proximity and there is less airflow. To place them outside is to risk them getting rained on.   I've heard of hikers finding unwanted guests in their boots in the morning. The thought of sticking my foot into my boot and finding a snake doesn't comfort me.

Fortunately Rex and I are on the shorter side and I can put our boots at the foot of our sleeping bags and on top of our packs. I'll clap off any excess dirt and place them up top. We've gotten used to the smell.... pretty much.

Your sense of smell sure does change. When we go past a tourist type area where there are a lot of day hikers, we are always amazed; they are so smelly! What is intended to be a sort of sport deodorant body-wash, or perfume, smells absolutely rancid. It is a sickingly sweet smell. I can smell a woman's hair spray from a good distance; rancid.

It makes me wonder how our pets can put up with us. We are all so excessively perfumed and stinky!

Below, Rex is soaking his legs. Also, bandanas are not just for hiker fashion. I have one tied under my nose. My nose runs nonstop in the cold weather. This keeps my nose warm.

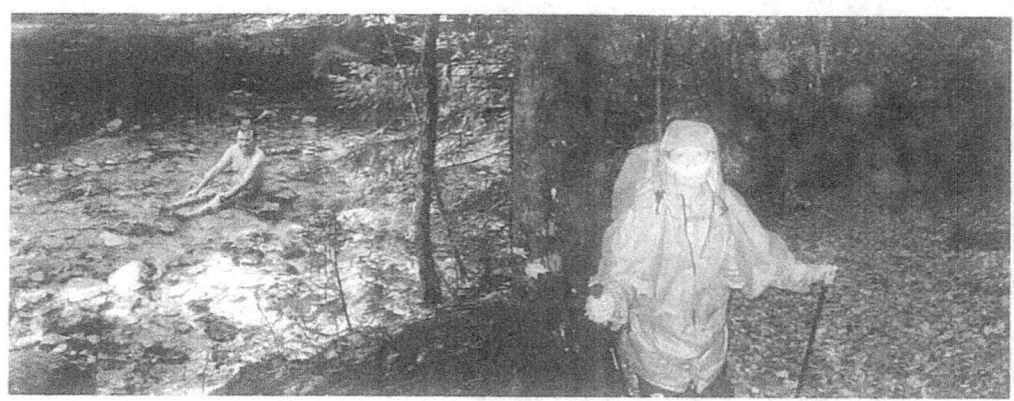

The dry spell has changed and we have been hiking thru the rain for days and Rex says that I can't take it out on him for the lousy weather. But he's the only one that I'm with and no one ever said "marriage would be fair"! I'm trying to remember that the bad times aren't his fault but sometimes I just can't stand it.

We spent a night at the Shook Branch Recreation Park in Hampton, TN. It is beautiful and we got some good pictures. It has bathrooms with running water even!

We stayed at the hostel "the Kincora" owned by Bob Peoples. Nice guy. He only charges $4. per night with laundry and shower. cool! We were bad company the night that we stayed there and went to bed early. While I lay in bed drifting off to sleep I enjoyed hearing Bob tell the other guests some of his stories. He is very good at story telling.

When we hiked up "the Priest" I was so tired of everyone telling us how bad it would be that I had a bit of an attitude (surprised?). I just kept hiking up and up, up, and I did wonder if I'd give myself another heart attack, until Rex asked me to stop for a minute. We laid down on a rock over-hang with our packs on for a moment before we continued forward. And then up up until we finally arrived at the shelter. We stopped and filled our water bottles and talked with other hikers for a minute and then set about putting up our tent and cooking. And along came "Red Wagon". I'll never forget that name. He presented to us the gift of a cold can of beer. WOW! He'd kept it cold in a stream. I took a sip but gave it to Rex to enjoy. What a kind gesture; a cold beer after hiking up to the top of a mountain was truly a surprise. It put a smile on my face. Thanks again Red Wagon!

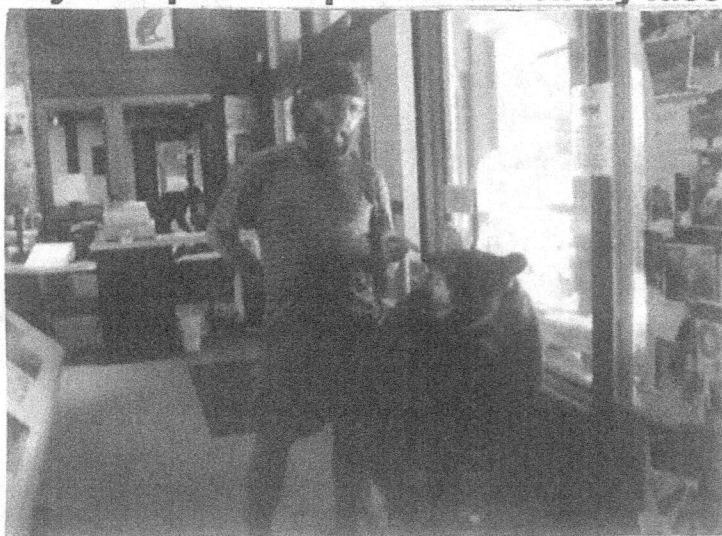

Stuffed bear at a
visitors center

We stayed at the Mountain Harbor Hostel in Roan Mountain, TN it was a short distance from the trail. We looked at the large home as we approached and it was beautiful with a stream running thru and horses and goats and a lovely porch around it and then I saw the barn and I said to Rex sarcastically "well, I know where I'll be sleeping tonight". Sure enough, the hikers were to stay in the barn. This barn was a far cry from the other barn type places we'd stayed. It was great inside! The upstairs is more like a bed and breakfast and I really didn't want to leave.

We stayed at another hostel. The owner was a chatter box. She was really very very nice. I just wanted food and sleep I wasn't feeling really talkative. Her neighbor was known to be crazy and was also known to yell at the hikers going past his house. He started his riding lawn mower and gunned the motor at 5am to make sure we were all up and awake and to complete the effect he flashed his head lights into the windows. I waved a big "hi" and smiled as he went past. I wanted to express my gratitude to him by trying to tell him we didn't oversleep.miserable bastard!

We stayed at Uncle Johnny's Hostel too and it was very cool. We were told about the towns history and about Mary the elephant. (I'll let you lookup this one) Someone told us that the town has roughly 5000 people and 600 churches . I thought that was a whole lot of churches and I said "Gee! can't they get along?"   ha ha

We could have avoided some of the hostels but we've heard so many stories about them that we would be missing out on part of "the trail experience" if we missed out on them.

We spent one night at a hotel also so that Rex could watch his Gators...big treat!

BEES

Rex has been stung 4 times; me only once. He hikes behind me and the bees get disturbed by me sometimes and he gets the brunt of it. When I got stung we were in town where I could put ice on it and keep my leg elevated and all and it wasn't a big deal.

There are sections of the trail that there is no other choice than to walk thru tall flowering weeds up above our heads. It made me nervous that I'd get stung and have an allergic reaction. I had only one epipen and hoped that we both wouldn't get stung. I tried to stay calm as not to attract any of the bees. I spent the whole time with my eyes darting back and forth across the trail looking for bees and moving aside branches quickly and gently with my hiking stick. Occasionally, holding one back for Rex to pass as well.

ANIMAL HUSBANDRY...

One day we are hiking along and I looked up from my boots and I said "good morning ladies" as I had seen cows. 'Those aren't cows" Rex said "they are bulls". I looked up again and looked at their under carriage and said "oh no they are bulls!". Well your most likely thinking these bulls are used to people hiking by them, right?

Well that reminds me of when a guy I knew from church who hosted a church picnic at his home, a farm. His normally docile bull charged a guest (this guest was an attorney no less). Well, the injured man went to the hospital and was found to have no bull-related injuries. They did however find something else, health wise, that needed tending to and it saved him great grief in the end.

And then there was this girl that got in a car accident and went to the hospital. The MRI of her head showed no car accident related injuries but it did show a brain tumor that she and her parents were real glad to be advised.

So sometimes bad things happen to save us from worse things. Is this part of why Rex and I had such a hard time getting back into the trail.; to save us from something worse?

So then the next day we are hiking along and I look up again and I said "oh no more bulls!", "no" Rex said "they are cows with horns". What! Again I looked at their undercarriage and thought "who keeps changing the rules?"

Leaves have been changing and falling since we've gotten back on the trail. They are really changing and falling now. In 3 days we will be coming thru the smokies. We've asked my step-mom to send our winter coats etc; yuck more weight. Keep us in your prayers please. I got some emails last time but have not yet responded. Please forgive me.

One last thing:

Another hiker asked me this:"have you heard about the woman that hiked the whole AT in 45 days?"

Knowing that the AT was being used merely as a racing/obstacle course, I said "yea.. but how much of the trail has she actually seen?!", and I was told "Well this is her third time doing it." "Well," I said sarcastically, "If she'd just slow down she'd only have to do it once!".

GOD BLESS!

This is one of my last big melt downs.

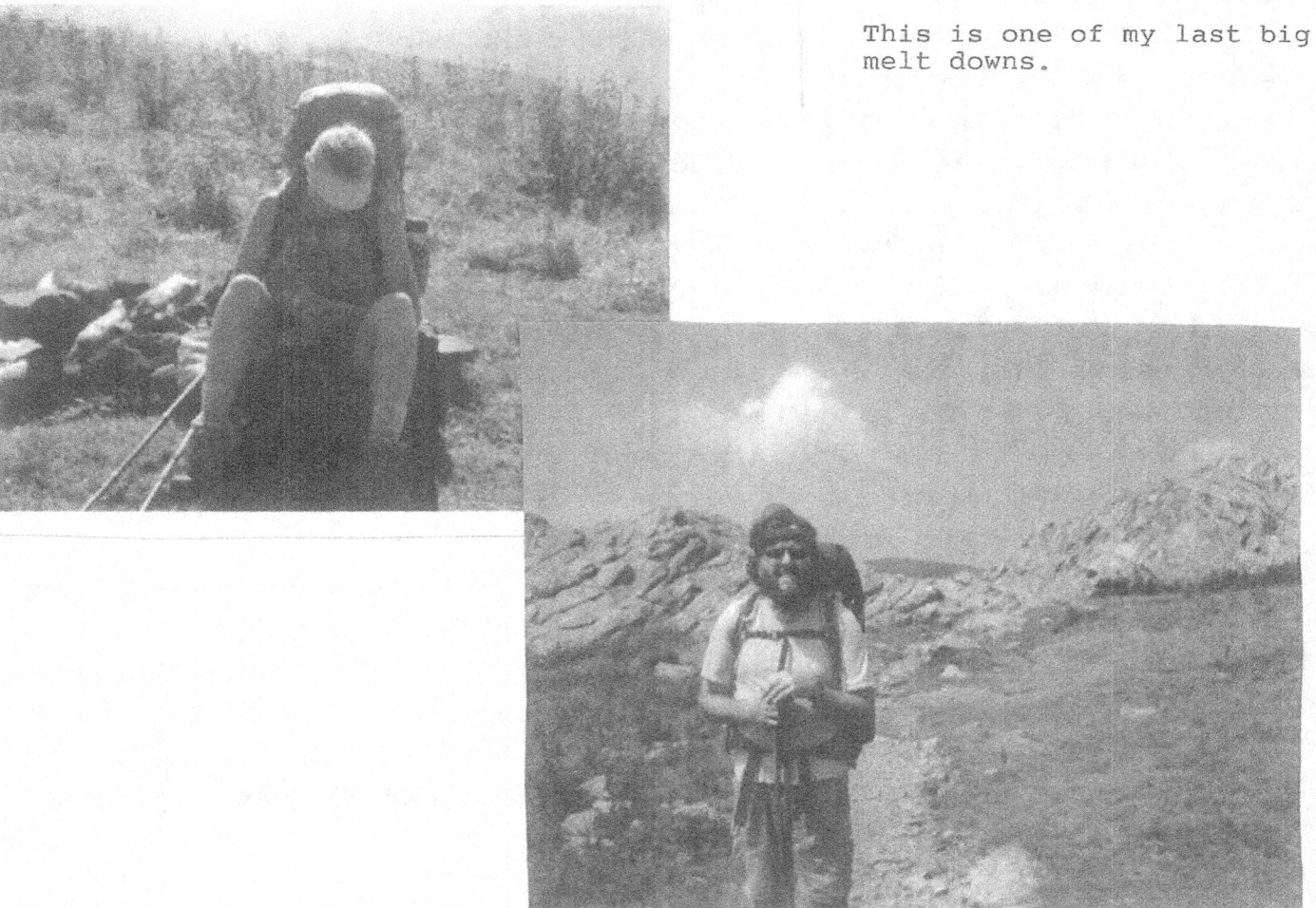

CHAPTER 9

We are in GATLINBURG, TN. and the count down is ...204.7 more miles to go to complete! It is very touristy here and we are having a ball with so many different eating options. We have decided to take a zero day and get fat and happy before moving forward. This may be our last good stop before we stop for good. We have been blessed with finding the GRAND PRIX MOTEL where the owner gives a special "hiker" rate of $29.99...clean sheets, bath with tub/shower, refrig., micro.. I've died and gone to heaven.

The stretch of Smokies that we have just come over was some of the best trail so far. The Smokie Mountain Parks trails have fairly easy "ups" compared to others that we have been on. To keep erosion to a minimum they have put loose rocks over the trails which is a common practice on the trail but it makes the hiking really difficult with your feet constantly shifting and slipping. It makes your knees and hips etc get real sore. But all together, going up from 1400 to 6360 feet could have been a whole lot more difficult. On the stretch into town the trail was fairly level with excellent views off either side of the trail. When I say "fairly level" I mean in an AT kind of a way.

Tomorrow we set off to go up and over Clingman's Dome. This is where Rex was inspired to do the trail when he and his family came thru the dome when he was about 12 years old. This is the highest part of the trail. As you may or may not know for every 1000 feet you go up.it gets cooler by 8 to 10 degrees and the leaves change about a week earlier for every 1000 feet. The next few days it is going to be freaky cold for us and it could be a record setter with the temperatures expecting to break a 1946 record. Perfect timing isn't it? So glad we asked my folks to send our winter coats, hats and gloves. I am over my little miserable spell. Mysteriously it seemed to go away with the rain. Now we are focusing on trying to complete the trail hopefully for Rex's birthday.

Just to make me feel bad, as I was complaining about the "young Hikers" and how they have a sense of entitlement etc. and my complaining about the weather and about the trail and about my feet/blisters and anything else that I could think of...we met a couple of younger hikers that totally put me to shame with their log book entries. They described how grateful they were to be doing the trail and how it was bringing them closer to God etc.

Don't you just hate that! Here I am having a well deserved "bitch session" and these kids come along all philosophical and spiritual and all and they make me look bad! Any way, with the end in sight now, I am enjoying the time we have left. Of course if I have cell phone reception on top of Clingman's Dome at night when it is freezing cold I may be singing a different tune. We are looking forward to getting back to our "normal" activities; Civil War Re enactments, my house cleaning business, but what is "normal" though? After all most of our married lives have been on the trail. more later. Keep us in your prayers..PLEASE!

****

We are still in Gatlinburg. We left yesterday to resume our trip. We hitched a ride back up to Newfound Gap in the back of a pick-up. As we were going up to the gap from roughly 1600 feet up to 5045 feet we noticed there were more clouds and the temperature was dropping quickly. When we got out of the truck it was soo windy but we thought that once we got in the woods we would have shelter from the wind. We hiked maybe 3/4 of a mile and I said to Rex that we would freeze that night! When he offered we could go back to Gatlinburg, I had to say yes. I was already freezing.

Usually the minute I start hiking I'm ready to start peeling off the clothes but not yesterday. We were told on the news that they were expecting a record to be broken from 1946. Soo, here we are still in Gatlinburg. This cold spell is expected to pass quickly.

When we were hiking back into town my ungloved thumb kept getting too cold and I'd have to switch hands. A couple stopped to give us a ride and they had just driven up to Clingman's Dome. The wife stayed in the car as the husband started to climb to the top. He got pelted by icy snow. He showed us pictures taken on his Blackberry and the trees were blowing and ice covered. I'm really glad we stopped! OFF tomorrow... back on the trail that is...pray for us!

We are in Hiawassee, GA.. Yes! We made it up and over Clingman's Dome and it was a beautiful day. This is where Rex was inspired to do the trail when he was just a boy. So, it was extra special for us.

When we were ascending we went past another hiker who was eating his lunch and when we were up top eating our lunch he came by and said that shortly after we'd passed him a bear came by. Darn; figures!

The next day we were hiking up a mountain (something new) and a hiker ahead of us stopped to tell us that he'd seen a cub go up a tree and he pointed out the cub to us. I was so excited! I saw what looked like a large squirrels nest up in the tree and when I looked to see better the cub shifted it's weight to get comfy and I saw it's ears and the outline of it's chubby little body. As I was moving closer in for an even better view Rex reminded me that Momma bear was most likely not too far away and we should keep going.

When we get into town we are told by the residents that the bears are coming down from the woods and into their trash etc. In Gatlinburg we were told that one night a bear was on the stairs of the visitors center!

Well all of the time that we'd lost in Gatlinburg got me rethinking the proposed daily milage that I'd come up with and I thought that if we pushed a little we could still make it to Springer for Rex's birthday. So we did 18 miles one night after getting back on the trail by hitching back up to Newfound Gap etc and came into the shelter area with our head lights on. We had peanut butter crackers and went to bed.

The next day we'd be on the trail early and if we could push a little more we could make it to the Fontana Dam Hilton; 23 miles away.

The Fontana Dam Hilton is a name that the hikers have lovingly called the shelter there because it has showers and is very fancy by hikers terms. Well we stopped for lunch at a shelter and got to talking to a section hiker and we still had 12 miles to go but I thought that it was time well spent to rest for a little bit. We got going again and stopped at a tenting spot and looked at the book. We had 5 or 7 miles more to go and it was starting to get a little dark. We figured we would pick up the pace and make it to the Hilton. Well I had figured that the miles into the Dam would be "tourist miles" but nothing was farther from the truth and we were hiking down a rocky trail and it was nasty! It was gettin dark and we pulled out our headlights. One wouldn't work so well. My back was aching. I've never had back problems before but my back killed me! Either the tent in my pack had shifted or I was trying to compensate for going around the corner in the same direction for so long but no matter. I was in a great deal of pain.

We stopped and I took off my pack and after a few moments I was better and set off again. Again I had to stop and take a break when the pain became unbearable. And after a half mile or so again I was in too much pain. I thought about all those that I know that have back problems and I could empathize. I sat down in the middle of the trail and took off my pack yet again. The thousand hikers before me must have all also stopped here; to pee! It stunk. We set off one more time and I couldn't go any further. And so at the next wide turn in the trail we set up our tent and went "to bed" with no dinner and we were all out of water, totally. We were thirsty and so close to the dam that we could see it's lights but we just couldn't get down to it. The trail was nasty and with one "good" head light it was slow going.

At 2:30 in the morning I woke up thirsty. Was it my imagination or were my eyes sinking into my head? I went back to sleep. In the morning my thirst situation actually felt better and I felt like we'd make it and so off we went. We made it down to the road. Where were the bloody blazes! It was hard enough to find them in the light of day! How could we have found them last night?

We made it to the visitor's center. What an extravagance! Stone tiled walls and floors with running water and PAPER TOWEL! I washed my hands and took off my "facial mask".

"What! you do spa treatments out on the trail?" you ask. Not really, but the sweat, runny nose stuff and spider webs make a kind of thin mask on your face. Great hu?

Rex said that we could spend the day at the Hilton and rest my back up. That's a great offer I thought, but it's cold outside and my back won't get better in the cold. So I called up the place where we were going to spend the next night to see if she did shuttles out to the dam as Rex was talking to the nice couple manning the visitor's center. Great! She'd be out to get us shortly.

The owner rented us a mini cabin. They call it a loft. It was a small cabin with a stack washer and dryer, a sink, a half bath, a TV! two twin beds..a micro. I was in heaven. We had our own heater. $30.00! What a great deal. I was tickled pink.

We did about 3 days of hiking after that stay with my back greatly improved and we got to the Nantahala Outdoor Center. This was a very touristy place and it was a weekend. I felt like an Amish person out of their culture. We looked and smelled different then the up scale people I saw.

We went to the store on the compound and they were all out of Ibuprofin. We got our "room key". What a "room key"? I thought this was just rows of bunks. We ate a surprisingly good dinner at the restaurant, even the kids portions were generous and looked good. And off to find our bunk house. When we opened our room I found what looked like a prison cell with it's having gray painted floors and gray painted wooden bench and two bunks. "Perfect" I said "just like home!" Not really, but I was giddy at the fact that we'd have a room to ourselves and we slept up on the full size bunk and used the lower twin size bed for our pack junk.

We left the N.O.C. and went straight up out of the gap from 1723 feet to over 5000 feet. I was getting really tired of this. I was getting really tired of this. Did I mention how tired of this I was getting? We got to Franklin, NC.. At first I didn't think that there was much business nearby the Budget Motel that we were staying at until we found the downtown. It was a short distance.

Making our way into town we saw some white blazes and then we noticed a sign for an outfitters. Great! We didn't even know that they were here!

We met the store owners with one of them being very pregnant. The other two owners were also very nice and we had a good time talking to them. We wished them much success.

We even got to take a peek in their history museum. This is something that we have done in quite a few of the towns that we've come through. If time permits etc we go and look around at whatever historical sites the town has to offer. It has surprised us what we have found.

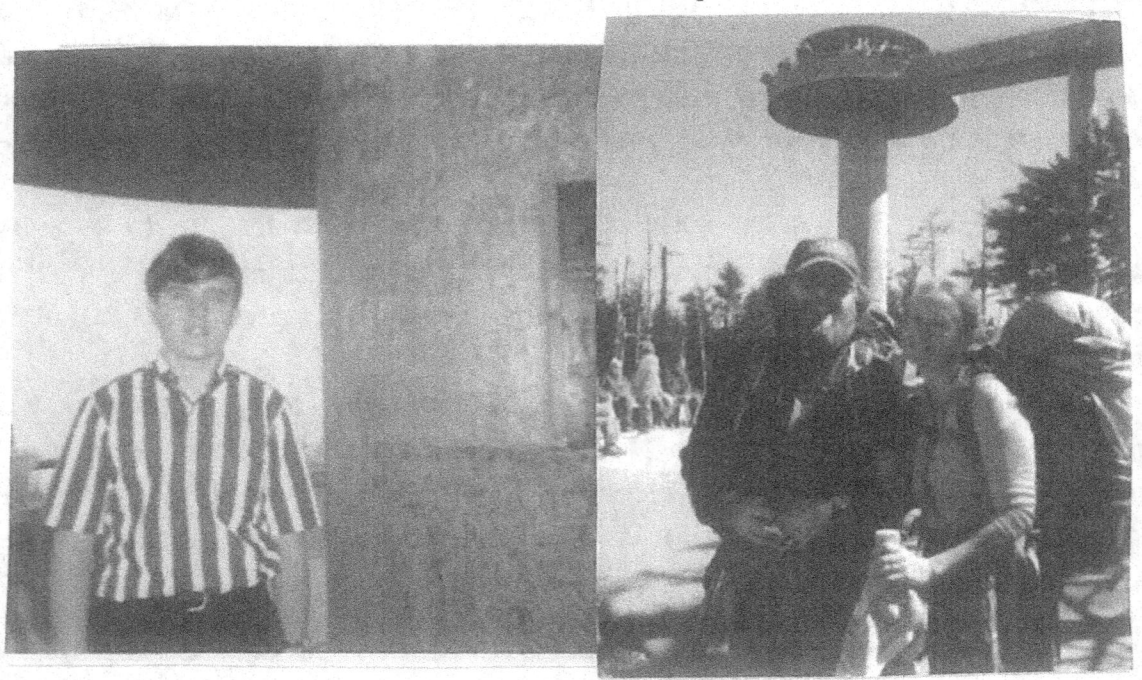

When Rex was 15 years old he and his family Visited Clingman's Dome. This is what inspired him.

In Pearisburg we toured a historical house. I can't wait to get back to Titusville and get involved in The Pritchard House there. Now we are in Hiawassee, GA. and it is Rex's birthday, October 15th. So much for finishing today. We only have about 6 more hiking days if I figure a special day for the last. We are at 67 miles and we are VERY excited. If all goes well we will only have a few miles to do on the last day to summit Springer Mountain.

Then we will hike down the approach trail to the visitor's center; basking in the glory and signing autographs with the TV crews taping the whole thing. (maybe..maybe not) Whatever! It will be a very big day for us.

Next stop will be Neel's Gap. If you've ever seen an AT video it's the place where the trail goes right thru the store and where all the north bounders (NOBOs) get new gear etc. That will be at mile marker 30.7 for us. Keep us in your prayers, as we do you. Not much further to go.

Oh yeah...MY FEET! We got me some new boots a few weeks ago and still blisters! Then I got some Keen's hiker sandals in Damascus. They did OK for a day or two and then you know what. So I was hiking around in those little black sandals. Then I figured a new way to secure the Keen's after the blisters had healed and we also got me some neoprene socks. The last few days...no blisters! FINALLY with less than 100 miles left to go I learn what to put on my feet!

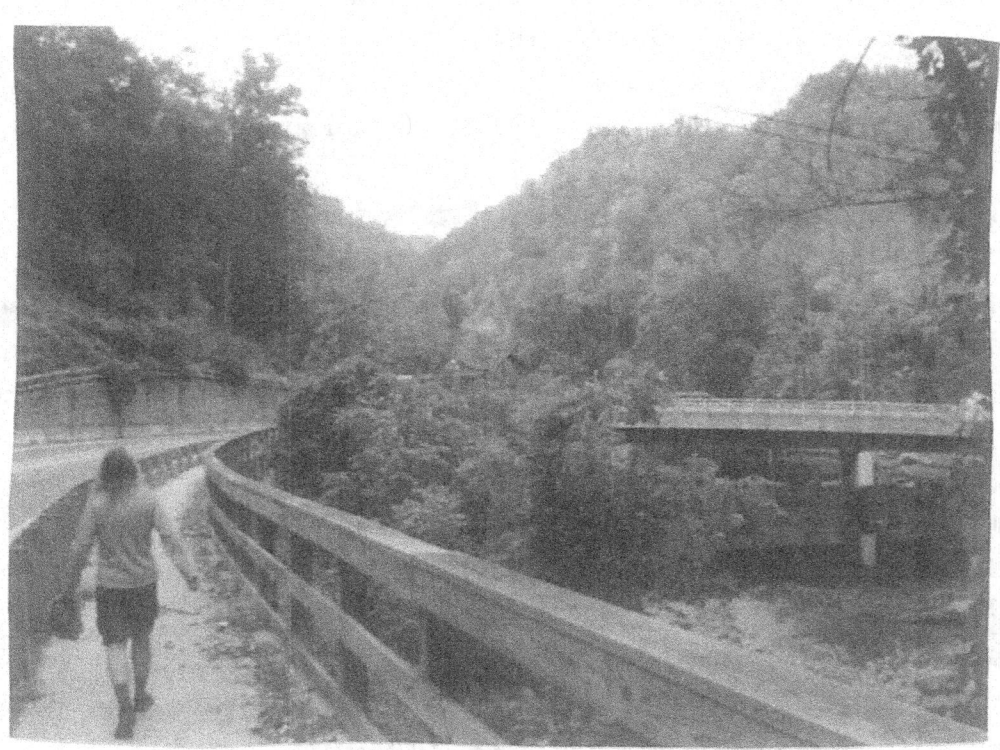

Colleen walking along the NOC.

CHAPTER 10

We left Hiawassee, GA late that day as we met up with Rex's long time friends Dan & Cindy. They had their Airstream camper in Helen, GA and we were going to hike 17 miles between Hiawassee and Helen and hitch over to their camp ground but the more I thought about it; how good of company would we be after doing 17 and then having to leave first thing in the morning.

So, we invited them to come visit us instead. It was real nice we'd never had "company" come visit while out on the trail. We have had quite a few good offers from people telling us about their family and close friends that we could call that would visit with us or help us in some way but it was always so hard to figure where we would be at what time. So I've just carried the names and numbers in case we got into a bind. So Dan & Cindy came and we got a good breakfast and they drove us to a pharmacy so that I could clean out the water bottles with hydrogen peroxide. Then they drove us back to the trail where I changed into my shorts and put on my Neoprene socks and then by the time it was time to say goodbye it was already time for me to get into some cooler socks.

The Neoprene socks are great in cold weather but other than they are hot. They don't keep your feet dry at all though they are just for warmth. If you walk thru a puddle you will feel what the temperature is of the water. It was hard to say goodbye....for me. It was crazy to think that we'd be hiking for hours nonstop. It still baffled my mind to think that we would hike for 8 to 10 hours a day.

It makes me think of the AT Trainer that Rex and I have thought up. You have a whole lot of time to think on the trail. It involves a sort of exercise unit that is simular to a treadmill but the walking surface keeps changing and the user would require an assistant. I'd recommend a teenager because they seem to be heartless and who would use things such as a water spray bottle and a fan. Or the assistant may drain out the water bottles and put a heat lamp on you. Of course there is the part of the training where the assistant rolls marbles and such under your feet. The possibilities of torture are endless.

Anyways, we stopped hiking after about 10 miles and the next day we hiked about 16 miles and the next day we hiked to a hostel as that night it was to rain hard. The hostel that we stayed at did not live up to the big hype that we'd seen on videos. It was obviously not during the big hiker season time when we got there. The staff seemed like they had had a bad busy season. Somehow I got it into my head that there was a restaurant nearby and there wasn't. I suppose that is my fault. We found there was a large refrigerator with frozen stuff, frozen hamburgs, pizza etc. So, we got a large supply of things to eat and our resupply and we paid for our bunks. I paid with our Visa. After I paid Rex realized that he wanted a drink. The drink was $1.70 for his modest sized drink; OK. Then we were informed that there was a minimum $5. purchase. What about all the money that I had just spent?!

We went to the bunk house and the refrigerator had locks on it. The computer was taken apart and put under a table. We were told that we hikers were not allowed to use the pizza oven. Someone would have to cook it for us because "we hikers" had proved ourselves to be un-trustworthy in the past.

The next morning we left late about 10am as we were letting the rain storm go past. So we set off into the rain and another couple headed in our direction came out after us and past us after a couple of hours. We stopped briefly on the trail and ate and drank a little. Then the couple came up behind us. We hadn't passed them. Had we? I figured that they were already at the next shelter because they seemed to be so much quicker that we were and we learned that they had stopped at a shelter in between to put on more clothing. They also said that the hostel where they were to stay after they made it to Springer said that they'd pick them up at the next gap if they wanted and that they should have cell phone coverage there. Would we like to join them?

It would be only 10 miles that we'd hike that day leaving 20 more to go. Well we'd already figured our miles to do 15 then 12.2 and the final 2. 8 miles on the last day with the 8.8 approach trail for the final day. I referred to it as our "glory day". We'd hike the final 2.8 miles and then sign autographs and answer questions for the news crews ha ha. So, this would mean that we'd hike 10 miles today and 17.2 tomorrow. "Sure" I said "this is our hike and we are doing it our way".

Then I thought, I should check with Rex! "Sure" he said. Great now I was in the lead as we all hiked to the gap to get picked up. I'd had Rex following me around for the length of the AT now I had this other couple who were faster hikers than I. Thank God the trail was pretty easy and I was able to go at a fairly good clip, for me anyways.

We got to the gap and they called for the ride and there was a group of people there that were also waiting for the same hostel to come get them as well. The weather was getting a little darker even though it was still very early and the wind was picking up and it was getting colder. Oh yea! I'm glad we are going indoors today. When the over sized van arrived we all squeezed in.

It was on of those times along the trail that I knew I'd miss. It was like we were a bunch of college kids or something although many were well over 50 years old. We laughed and joked and were so grateful to be going indoors for the night.

We got to the hostel and it was beautiful. It was an over sized log home that was still very new and we were assigned where we would sleep. Because there were two of us couples and quite a few older women; the women got the traditional bunk area and ourselves and the other couple were assigned private rooms with private baths. WOW! Are you serious!

"How much is this going to cost us?" Rex asked. "does it matter? " I asked. "No, not really!" he replied. The hostel was $18. per person and hopefully we still qualified for that rate.

The hostel owners kitchen on the main floor was off limits to hikers due to health Dept. rules but the lower level had a complete kitchen that we could use. We were offered the option to get a fancy coffee made by our guests for a nominal fee. "A decaf coffee for Rex and I'd like a hot chocolate." I asked.

What a nice place this was! Upon checking out in the morning we were just charged $44. This included the extras.

The next day was very cool. I was trying to savor every moment because the miles were definitely numbered now. We set up our tent inside the shelter with only 2.8 miles left to go in the morning. The other hikers staying there that night were very nice.

The other couple, who were to complete the end of the trail the next day, left most of their pack weight with the hostel owners and slackpacked to the top of Spring Mountain. They knew that they could easily do the 20 miles with no pack weight. They had a wedding to go to in a few days with many things left to do beforehand.

Rex and I ate Ramen noodles for one last time on that last night. (Every year on our AT anniversary I plan to serve him Ramen Noodles.)

We got up and were out by 8:17 the next morning. We easily hiked up to our destination. It made me think of when you give a dog a steak before putting him down! It was too easy. It was great.

We'd worked so hard and did truly deserve an easy finish. I needed one. I was done. I was finished. I had enough.

We celebrated with a couple that we met along the way. They graciously took our picture and celebrated with us. I'd like to see them again. They are from Tallahassee, FL..

Next we had the 8.8 hike down to the visitors center. I wasn't looking forward to this all together. I liked it in idea but I was tired. We informed everyone that we met along the way that we had just completed the AT in it's entirety. Some were impressed and I think a few thought that we were bragging. Who knows? It was our day and we were enjoying it.

We came down the falls and it was beautiful and I was enjoying this "glory time" that we had. We came thru the archway to the visitors center....just like Rex had always pictured.

We did this hike OUR WAY. South bounders, no flip flopping direction, no slack packing, and no blue blazing. This is how Rex defined how he wanted his hike to go. There is nothing wrong with doing it another way but this is how Rex wanted His hike to go. It was a glorious day and the weather was with us giving us a nice sunny slightly cool day. We were home. (almost)

After some bbq on the way home we got back to my folk's house late that night. On Sunday we headed to Rex's brothers and the next morning back to Titusville.

Today is Tues. Nov. 1st. Rex and I are at my folks house. We got off trail Friday afternoon Oct. 21st and we have been busy ever since. The last 60 something miles I won't soon forget.

I'd called my cleaning customers and everyone wanted me back right away. I had work the next day after we'd gotten home then thru to Friday. Yippi! Not only do we greatly need the money but it was reassuring that my customers still wanted me.

Being home with out work makes me depressed. I am much better off to stay busy.

God has blessed us in so many ways. Going back on and off the trail has been good for us as a couple. When we could come home I'd do something to the house that made it feel more mine too.

Usually, this involves Rex's stuff displayed my way. We have fast forwarded our relationship in unbelievable ways. We are no longer are embarrassed to fart in front of each other for one thing. ha ha

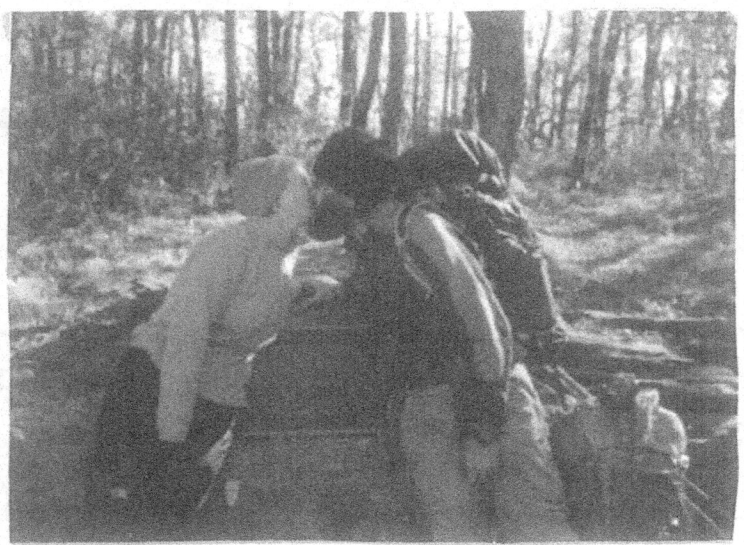

Yippi!   We made it!

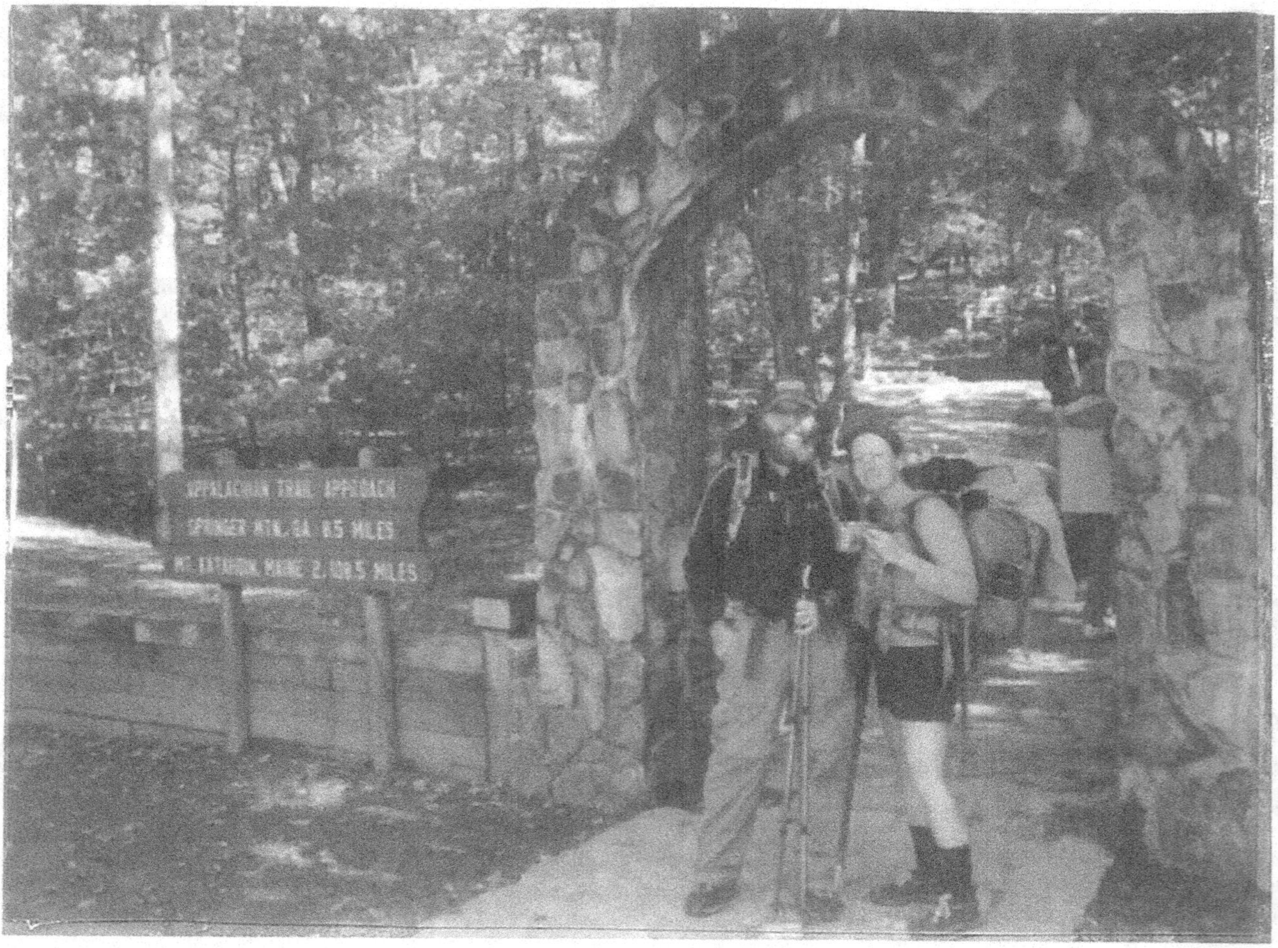

So what will we do with the millions of dollars we make from the sale of this book?

First off, I'm not really expecting to make *quite* that much. We will pay off our hiker debt.

Any excess money we will use to help us finance the Appalachian Trail Presentations that we do. We don't get paid for these and we could use a little gas money and money to help us provide Trail Magic to our guests.

Any more funds and we'll be raising Alpacas in North Carolina. No, I'm not kidding.

And finally, any larger funds and I will become involved in a charity so that I might answer some of the larger callings of my soul.

If the unlikely should happen, and we do not make millions or even hundreds, WELL, who cares! The fact that I have completed this book is enough. Rex and I will continue to do our presentations and encourage others to do "their AT".

What is your AT?

Tonight Rex and family are watching football and I am going to try and get some fishing line thread thru a spot on Rex's boot that has made a little hole on the side.

That's it for now folks....

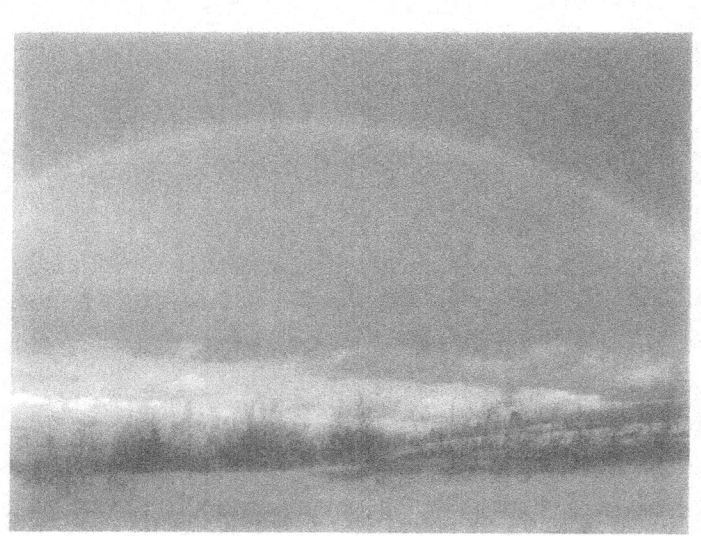

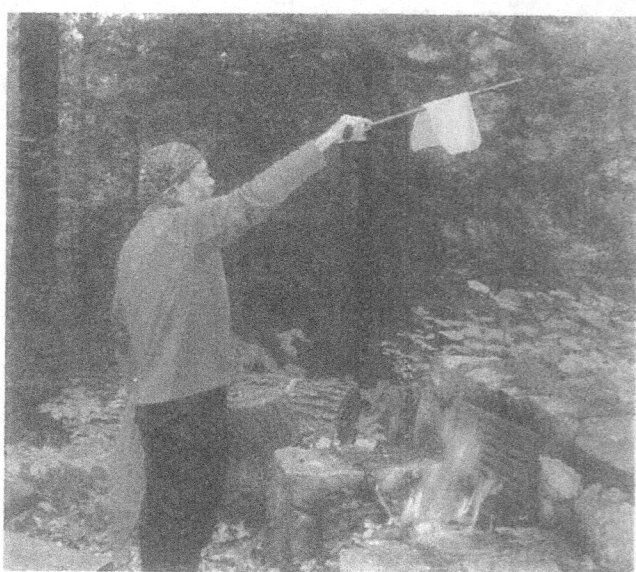

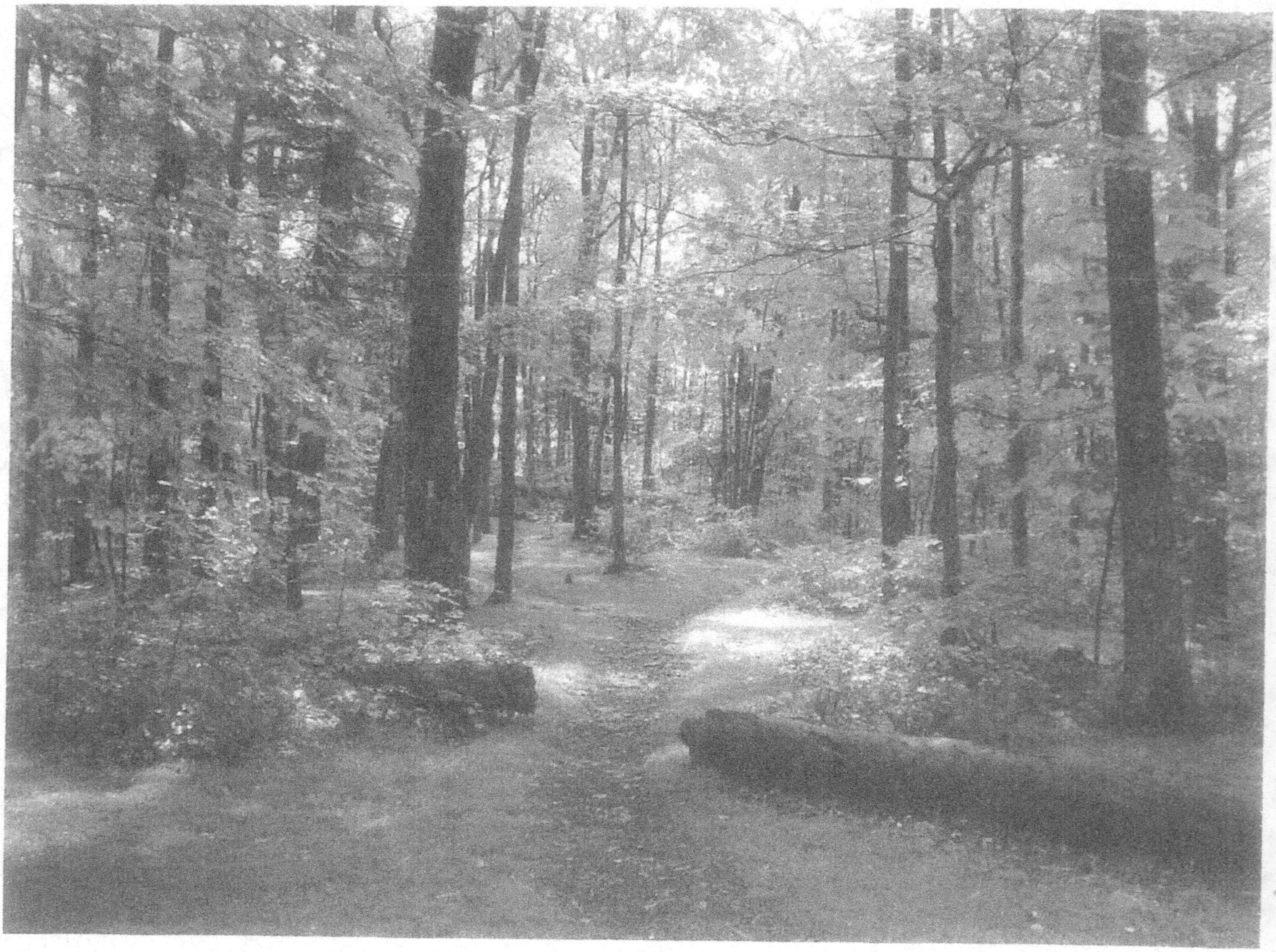

www.ingramcontent.com/pod-product-compliance
Lightning Source LLC
Chambersburg PA
CBHW081109290526
45795CB00006B/2055